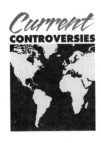

Current
CONTROVERSIES

Resistant Infections

Other Books in the Current Controversies Series

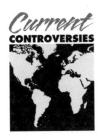

Current
CONTROVERSIES

Resistant Infections

Debra A. Miller, Book Editor

GREENHAVEN PRESS
A part of Gale, Cengage Learning

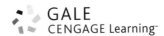

GALE
CENGAGE Learning™

Detroit • New York • San Francisco • New Haven, Conn • Waterville, Maine • London

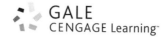

Christine Nasso, *Publisher*
Elizabeth Des Chenes, *Managing Editor*

© 2009 Greenhaven Press, a part of Gale, Cengage Learning

Gale and Greenhaven Press are registered trademarks used herein under license.

For more information, contact:
Greenhaven Press
27500 Drake Rd.
Farmington Hills, MI 48331-3535
Or you can visit our Internet site at gale.cengage.com

Articles in Greenhaven Press anthologies are often edited for length to meet page requirements. In addition, original titles of these works are changed to clearly present the main thesis and to explicitly indicate the author's opinion. Every effort is made to ensure that Greenhaven Press accurately reflects the original intent of the authors. Every effort has been made to trace the owners of copyrighted material.

Cover image copyright Michael Taylor, 2009. Used under license from Shutterstock.com.

LIBRARY OF CONGRESS CATALOGING-IN-PUBLICATION DATA

Resistant infections / Debra A. Miller, book editor.
p. cm. -- (Current controversies)
Includes bibliographical references and index.
ISBN 978-0-7377-4464-4 (hardcover)
ISBN 978-0-7377-4465-1 (pbk.)
1. Drug resistance. 2. Drug resistance in microorganisms. I. Miller, Debra A.
QR177.R467 2009
616.9'041--dc22

2009016633

Printed in the United States of America
1 2 3 4 5 6 7 13 12 11 10 09

Contents

Chapter 2: Are Drug-Resistant Infections the Result of Agricultural Use of Antibiotics?

No: The Rise of Drug-Resistant Infections Is Not the Result of Agricultural Use of Antibiotics

Chapter 3: Are Drug Companies at Fault for Not Developing Better Antibacterial Drugs?

Yes: The Drug Companies Are at Fault for Failing to Develop Better Antibacterial Drugs

Foreword

By definition, controversies are "discussions of questions in which opposing opinions clash" (Webster's Twentieth Century Dictionary Unabridged). Few would deny that controversies are a pervasive part of the human condition and exist on virtually every level of human enterprise. Controversies transpire between individuals and among groups, within nations and between nations. Controversies supply the grist necessary for progress by providing challenges and challengers to the status quo. They also create atmospheres where strife and warfare can flourish. A world without controversies would be a peaceful world; but it also would be, by and large, static and prosaic.

The Series' Purpose

The purpose of the Current Controversies series is to explore many of the social, political, and economic controversies dominating the national and international scenes today. Titles selected for inclusion in the series are highly focused and specific. For example, from the larger category of criminal justice, Current Controversies deals with specific topics such as police brutality, gun control, white collar crime, and others. The debates in Current Controversies also are presented in a useful, timeless fashion. Articles and book excerpts included in each title are selected if they contribute valuable, long-range ideas to the overall debate. And wherever possible, current information is enhanced with historical documents and other relevant materials. Thus, while individual titles are current in focus, every effort is made to ensure that they will not become quickly outdated. Books in the Current Controversies series will remain important resources for librarians, teachers, and students for many years.

In addition to keeping the titles focused and specific, great care is taken in the editorial format of each book in the series. Book introductions and chapter prefaces are offered to provide background material for readers. Chapters are organized around several key questions that are answered with diverse opinions representing all points on the political spectrum. Materials in each chapter include opinions in which authors clearly disagree as well as alternative opinions in which authors may agree on a broader issue but disagree on the possible solutions. In this way, the content of each volume in Current Controversies mirrors the mosaic of opinions encountered in society. Readers will quickly realize that there are many viable answers to these complex issues. By questioning each author's conclusions, students and casual readers can begin to develop the critical thinking skills so important to evaluating opinionated material.

Current Controversies is also ideal for controlled research. Each anthology in the series is composed of primary sources taken from a wide gamut of informational categories including periodicals, newspapers, books, U.S. and foreign government documents, and the publications of private and public organizations. Readers will find factual support for reports, debates, and research papers covering all areas of important issues. In addition, an annotated table of contents, an index, a book and periodical bibliography, and a list of organizations to contact are included in each book to expedite further research.

Perhaps more than ever before in history, people are confronted with diverse and contradictory information. During the Persian Gulf War, for example, the public was not only treated to minute-to-minute coverage of the war, it was also inundated with critiques of the coverage and countless analyses of the factors motivating U.S. involvement. Being able to sort through the plethora of opinions accompanying today's major issues, and to draw one's own conclusions, can be a complicated and frustrating struggle. It is the editors' hope that Current Controversies will help readers with this struggle.

Introduction

"Methicillin-resistant Staphylococcus au-reus, *or MRSA, is spreading rapidly throughout the population and has now become the poster child for an emerging crisis of antibiotic-resistant infections, both in the United States and around the world."*

Staphylococcus aureus, often simply called staph, is a type of bacteria that lives on the skin or in the nasal passages of 25 to 30 percent of all healthy people in the United States. For most people, these bacteria cause no problems or illness. But a hardy strain of the staph bacteria has developed a resistance to the traditional staph treatment of methicillin, a penicillin-related antibiotic, and this more dangerous type of staph can cause serious infection or even death. Indeed, methicillin-resistant *Staphylococcus aureus*, or MRSA, is spreading rapidly throughout the population and has now become the poster child for an emerging crisis of antibiotic-resistant infections, both in the United States and around the world.

MRSA often has been called the "flesh-eating bacteria" in news reports, but this is a misnomer because the bacteria really do not eat flesh; instead, the bacteria releases toxins that cause body tissues to break down. Infection may begin with a red spot on the skin that looks like a pimple, a boil, or a spider bite. In many cases, the boil will rupture and drain, and then resolve itself without any need for medical intervention. And even for the vast majority of people afflicted with MRSA who must seek medical help, the bacteria produce only minor skin infections that are easily treated with certain powerful antibiotics. But because MRSA can be detected only by a skin culture that takes days to be assessed by a laboratory, doctors in the meantime often prescribe ineffective antibiotics, sometimes allowing painful skin infections to linger, recur, or spread for days or weeks, creating long recovery periods and great frustration for some patients. In addition, MRSA is highly communicable, and infected people who are not properly treated can easily transmit the infection to their families, coworkers, or school classmates.

The worst outcomes of a MRSA infection, however, come when the infection does not attack the skin, but other parts of the body. In relatively rare instances, MRSA can lead to life-threatening conditions such as infections of the bloodstream or heart valves, toxic shock syndrome, and pneumonia. Tragically, the victims of these more serious types of MRSA often are young and otherwise very healthy. One recent victim, for example, was 20-year-old Chris Fenden, a student from Western Washington University. After two weeks of suffering from a lingering cough, Chris's condition worsened. He went to the school health center on a Thursday night, February 14, 2008, complaining of flu-like symptoms—fever, vomiting, and coughing up blood. He was immediately taken to a local hospital and placed in intensive care, but it was too late for antibiotics to work. Chris died the following Wednesday from pneumonia caused by MRSA.

MRSA first emerged in the 1960s in hospitals and other health care settings, where it often spread easily among post-surgery and intensive care patients who had open wounds, required body-invasive procedures such as ventilators or catheters, or who were older people with weak or compromised immune systems. A recent study by the Association for Professionals in Infection Control and Epidemiology, for example, found that 46 of every 1,000 hospital patients in the United States develop MRSA infections. The high incidence of MRSA infections in hospitals has led many hospitals to take much stricter precautions, such as requiring more frequent hand-washing and other hygiene efforts, testing for MRSA, and mandating careful sanitation of areas contaminated by MRSA patients. Thanks to these actions, the U.S. Centers for Disease Control and Prevention (CDC)—the nation's top public health agency—has reported that the rate of MRSA infections among intensive care unit patients in U.S. hospitals has declined during the past five years.

Yet even as hospitals seem to have some success in controlling MRSA, the MRSA threat is becoming increasingly common in community settings. Although most community cases are skin infections, severe and often fatal cases of MRSA-caused pneumonia and other conditions continue to occur. Outbreaks of MRSA have occurred in families and among athletes, prisoners, members of the military, children in daycare, and other places where people live in crowded conditions or share bathrooms, sports equipment, or other items. These community-based MRSA bacteria now cause 95,000 serious infections and 20,000 deaths every year in the United States.

Perhaps the most frightening aspect of the MRSA story, however, is that experts fear that some community-acquired MRSA strains are developing into "superbugs"—bacteria that can resist not only penicillin-based antibiotics but also a wide range of other antibiotics that used to be effective against MRSA. A recent CDC study, for example, found that 10 percent of the common community strains of MRSA are now resistant to non-penicillin antibiotics such as clindamycin, tetracycline, and Bactrim. In addition, the superbug MRSA strains, when they invade hospitals, seem to be able to swap gene components with other bacteria to become even more drug resistant. One antibiotic, vancomycin, is now considered the drug of last resort against the most virulent strains of MRSA, but if it becomes ineffective, there may be no way to stop the spread of MRSA. Many doctors think MRSA is poised to become a major epidemic, both in the United States and in other countries.

But MRSA is only one of a number of types of bacteria that are becoming resistant to antibiotic drugs. Other types of drug-resistant bacteria that concern health officials in the United States include *Streptococcus pneumonia* (another type of bacteria that causes pneumonia), *Enterococcus faecium* (a highly drug resistant bacteria that can cause abdominal, skin, urinary tract, and blood infections), and gram-negative bacilli (a group of bacteria that can cause serious conditions such as sexually transmitted gonorrhea, meningitis, and respiratory disease). In addition, one in seven new cases of tuberculosis, or TB, is drug-resistant; this and a number of other drug-resistant diseases are already causing millions of deaths in the developing world.

Scientists say the development of drug-resistant strains of bacteria is not surprising, because it is natural for bacteria to evolve in ways that will eventually produce resistance to various drugs. Yet many experts say the problem has become a crisis largely due to human factors, such as poor hygiene habits in health care settings, the overuse of antibiotic drugs in medicine, the practice of feeding antibiotics to animals grown for food, and the reluctance of major drug companies to develop new antibiotic drugs. Proposed solutions seek to correct one or more of these causal factors. The viewpoints included in *Current Controversies: Resistant Infections* explore these and other questions central to this important issue.

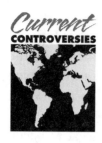

CHAPTER 1

How Serious Is the Problem of Resistant Infections?

Chapter Overview

Teddi Dineley Johnson

Teddi Dineley Johnson is a reporter for The Nation's Health, *which is the official monthly newspaper of the American Public Health Association.*

With American wallets getting tighter, loosening the price tag on prescription drugs commonly used by consumers is becoming a growing trend among U.S. pharmacies and stores—including new offers for free antibiotics at grocery stores. But with antibiotic-resistant infections on the rise, public health experts warn that "free" can come at a dangerously high price.

In January [2009], several major grocery store chains announced plans to give free generic antibiotics to customers with valid prescriptions. Through March [2009], shoppers can present prescriptions to receive free, 14-day supplies of commonly prescribed antibiotics such as amoxicillin, penicillin and tetracycline. But while the promise of free antibiotics may entice cost-cutting consumers, it is raising alarm bells for many in public health, especially those who have been working to combat misuse of antibiotics.

Promoting free antibiotics at a time when the nation faces a growing crisis of antibiotic resistance "does not make good public health sense," according to the Infectious Diseases Society of America, which criticized the giveaways.

"Most doctors know better than to prescribe antibiotics when they are not needed," said Anne Gershon, MD, president of the Infectious Diseases Society of America. "But many find it hard to say 'no' to sick patients who think antibiotics will

Teddi Dineley Johnson, "Free Offers of Antibiotics Raise Concern for Some in Public Health," *The Nation's Health*, vol. 39, March 2009, pp. 1, 14. Copyright © 2009 *The Nation's Health*. Reproduced by permission.

21

make them feel better. We are concerned that these pharmacy marketing efforts will encourage patients to ask for antibiotics prescriptions."

Antibiotic Resistance Is a Threat

Antibiotic resistance is "one of the key microbial threats to health in the United States," according to the Institute of Medicine, which has recommended curbing the inappropriate use of antibiotics—such as using them for illnesses they do not treat, like colds or the flu, or using them to enhance growth among livestock.

Unfortunately, antibiotic resistance has been growing in recent decades, making it harder to treat infectious diseases such as tuberculosis and methicillin-resistant Staphylococcus aureus, or MRSA. According to the Centers for Disease Control and Prevention [CDC], MRSA caused more than 94,000 life-threatening infections in the United States in 2005. Multidrug-resistant TB is a growing threat around the world, and recent reports have documented drug resistance among Clostridium difficile, a bacteria that can cause serious intestinal conditions. Compounding the issue is that few new antibiotics are being developed to replace those that are losing effectiveness.

The free antibiotic offers are dangerous because they could lead consumers to stockpile the drugs, John Santa, MD, MPH, director of the Consumer Reports Health Rating Center, told *The Nation's Health.* Consumers could meet with more than one doctor, get multiple prescriptions and save the antibiotics for later "and that is not a trend we want to encourage or facilitate these days," Santa said.

Another concern is that when antibiotics are free, patients want them even more, Santa said, noting that during more than 20 years as a primary care internist, situations involving patients demanding antibiotics were one of the most challenging for him.

"It is frustrating for practicing physicians to see that major chains are reinforcing that behavior rather than discouraging it," he said.

In some cases, advertisements being used to hype the free antiobiotic campaigns are misleading, said Ed Septimus, MD, a member of the board of directors of the Infectious Diseases Society of America, who noted that some of the ads tout the free antibiotics as coming just in time for winter colds and flu.

We want to make sure that when [antibiotics] are being used, they are being used appropriately.

"These conditions are primarily viral, so they are giving the wrong message to the public that somehow flu and cold and cough should be treated with antibiotics," Septimus told *The Nation's Health*. "There is significant literature that suggests that the majority of these prescriptions are inappropriate for upper respiratory infections, most of them being viral. So our concern regarding a program like this is that we don't want to put any additional pressure, both on consumers and prescribers, to prescribe unnecessary antibiotics."

How to Appropriately Use Antibiotics

Public health organizations and advocates have been actively working in past decades to educate both consumers and physicians on the safe use of antibiotics and have been making inroads.

CDC's "Get Smart: Know When Antibiotics Work" campaign teaches how to reduce resistance brought on by overuse and over-prescribing of antibiotics. The program's goal is to build consumers' and health care providers' awareness about appropriate antibiotic use, said the campaign's director, Lauri Hicks, DO. Studies have shown that such efforts can be effective.

To combat the message that may be conveyed by the grocery store freebies, Hicks said CDC and the Infectious Diseases Society of America will ask retailers that offer free antibiotics to partner with the Get Smart program and distribute materials to their customers on inappropriate antibiotic use.

"We don't want to limit access to people that actually do need them," she said. "We want to make sure that when they are being used, they are being used appropriately."

Jamie Miller, spokesman for Maryland-based Giant Food, which is one of the grocery stores offering the free antibiotics, told *The Nation's Health* that the company is "open to listening to what constituents and government agencies may want to talk to us about." Giant's free antibiotic program is designed for customers who have been prescribed antibiotics by their physicians, "who have an obligation to look out for the safety and well-being of their customers," he said.

Providing free medicine may get customers into stores, said Septimus, of the Infectious Diseases Society of America. But a more responsible marketing effort would be to offer free flu shots, he said.

"If you can prevent an infection like influenza, which we know is associated with significant mortality and morbidity, it would be much more beneficial to the community to offer free flu vaccines than offering free antibiotics," Septimus said.

Antibiotic-Resistant Infections Are an Epidemic in the United States and Worldwide

Brad Spellberg, Robert Guidos, David Gilbert, John Bradley, Helen W. Boucher, W. Michael Scheld, John G. Bartlett, and John Edwards, Jr.

Brad Spellberg is an assistant professor of medicine at the David Geffen School of Medicine at the University of California Los Angeles. Robert Guidos is the director of Public Policy and Government Relations at the Infectious Diseases Society of America. David Gilbert, John Bradley, Helen W. Boucher, W. Michael Scheld, John G. Bartlett, and John Edwards, Jr. are infectious disease researchers from various universities located throughout the United States.

We are in the midst of an emerging crisis of antibiotic resistance for microbial pathogens in the United States and throughout the world. Epidemic antibiotic resistance has been described in numerous pathogens in varying contexts, including—but not limited to—a global pandemic of methicillin-resistant *Staphylococcus aureus* (MRSA) infection; the global spread of drug resistance among common respiratory pathogens, including *Streptococcus pneumoniae* and *Mycobacterium tuberculosis*, and epidemic increases in multidrug-resistant (and, increasingly, truly pan-resistant) gram-negative bacilli. Infections caused by these and other antibiotic-resistant microbes impact clinicians practicing in every field of medicine. Given their breadth of effect and significant impact on morbidity and mortality, multidrug-resistant microbes are considered a substantial threat to US public health and national security by the National Academy of Science's Institute of Medicine, the federal Interagency Task Force on Antimicrobial Resistance (Interagency Task Force), and the Infectious Diseases Society of America (IDSA). . . .

What Is the Cause of Antibiotic Resistance?

In the aftermath of the unprecedented successes of early antibiotic therapies, in the late 1960s, US Surgeon General William H. Stewart is alleged to have made the now infamous declaration that "[it] is time to close the book on infectious diseases and declare the war against pestilence won". Although this statement may well be apocryphal, it clearly reflects the general sentiment in the medical community at the time. Unfortunately, the past 30 years have revealed how grossly inaccurate that sentiment was. Indeed, we are further away than ever from "closing the book on infectious diseases," which, despite the availability of antibiotics, remain the second-leading cause of death worldwide and the third-leading cause of death in the United States.

The global spread of microbial resistance is a predominant reason why infectious diseases have not been conquered. It is commonly expressed that physician misuse of antibiotics is the cause of antibiotic resistance in microbes and that, if we could only convince physicians to use antibiotics responsibly, we could "win the war against microbes." Unfortunately, this belief is a fallacy that reflects an alarming lack of respect for the incredible power of microbes.

As diverse as human beings are, we pale in comparison with the adaptability of microbes, which inhabit literally every possible climate and environment on the planet, despite extremes of boiling or freezing temperatures, pressures sufficient to crush virtually any human-made submersible, extreme salinity, zero oxygen content, presence or absence of sunlight, etc. Indeed, from the microbial perspective, human beings are nothing more than walking microbial planets; there are 5–10 times more microbes living on and in every human being than there are human cells in our bodies. Bacteria even exist in large numbers miles deep in the midst of solid rock in the earth's crust. Because of this extraordinary diversity of habitat, microbes comprise fully 60% of the biomass on the planet (90% if cellulose is excluded from the calculation), despite their submicron size.

Microbes have had 3.5 billion years to adapt to the various environments on planet Earth. The power that drives microbial adaptability is genetic plasticity and rapid replication. It takes many bacteria only 20–30 minutes to replicate; it takes human beings 20–30 years to replicate. Given the above, there is no doubt that microbes are the most numerous, diverse, and adaptable organisms that have ever lived on the planet.

Human beings ... [encourage bacterial resistance with] the thousands of metric tons of antibiotics we have used in patients and livestock over the past half century.

On reflection, perhaps it would be wise to reconsider the frequently used metaphor of humans being "at war with microbes". It is absurd to believe that we could ever claim victory in a war against organisms that outnumber us by a factor of 10^{22}, that outweigh us by a factor of 10^8, that have existed for 1,000 times longer than our species, and that can undergo as many as 500,000 generations during 1 of our generations. Furthermore, the weapons in a war against microbes would be antibiotics. We need to remember that human beings did not invent antibiotics; we merely discovered them. Genetic analysis of microbial metabolic pathways indicates that microbes invented both β-lactam antibiotics and β-lactamase enzymes to resist those antibiotics > [more than] 2 billion years ago. In contrast, antibiotics were not discovered by humans until the first half of the 20th century. Thus, microbes have had collective experience creating and defeating antibiotics for 20 million times longer than *Homo sapiens* have known that antibiotics existed.

Ultimately, we must concede that we will never truly defeat microbial resistance; we can only keep pace with it.

The Human Factor

From this framework, it is obvious that microbes do not need our help in creating antibiotic resistance. On the other hand, what human beings can do is affect the rate of spread of bacterial resistance by applying selective pressure via exposure to the thousands of metric tons of antibiotics we have used in patients and livestock over the past half century. Methods to control unnecessary use of antibiotics include appropriate regulations on use of antibiotics in agriculture (including elimination of use of antibiotics to promote growth of food animals), restriction of antibiotic use to pathogen-specific agents, and limits on the common practice of using antibacterial agents for viral infections. Clearly, it is desirable to use antibiotics only when appropriate, to try to limit selective pressure that increases the frequency of resistance. Nevertheless, the distinction between causality of microbial resistance and the rate of spread of resistance must be recognized if we are to create a true solution to the problem of antibiotic resistance. If our misuse of antibiotics causes drug resistance, the solution that would allow us to forever defeat microbial resistance would be for us to strictly use antibiotics only when truly indicated. On the other hand, if our misuse of antibiotics affects the rate of spread of resistance but does not actually cause resistance, then using antibiotics correctly will not stop microbial resistance, it will only slow it down so that we can find a real solution to the problem. Framed in this context, it is clear that convincing physicians to use antibiotics properly is an important step to take, not because it is a solution to drug resistance, but because it will buy us more time to create a real solution to the problem.

Antimicrobial effectiveness is a precious, limited resource. Therefore, preserving antibiotic effectiveness can be viewed similar to society's responses to overconsumption and depletion of other precious, limited resources, such as oil and other energy sources, clean water and air, and forests. When supply of these other resources has been threatened, society has stepped in to protect them from further consumption/depletion (e.g., energy conservation and restrictions on factory pollution) and to promote their restoration (e.g., forest restoration). Here, the resource that must be protected and restored is antibiotic "effectiveness." Society has tried to protect this resource against depletion through antimicrobial stewardship, including the placement of appropriate restrictions on antibiotic use, and through infection control. Unfortunately, society has not acted to promote antibiotic restoration (i.e., the development of new antibiotics), and antibiotic restrictions have the unintended, negative consequence of further destabilizing an already fragile market situation for antibiotic R&D [research and development].

Ultimately, we must concede that we will never truly defeat microbial resistance; we can only keep pace with it. The only viable, long-term solution to the problem of microbial resistance is to have in place in perpetuity a continuing, steady development of new antibiotics and other strategies (including immunotherapeutics and vaccines, diagnostics and antibiotic stewardship programs to improve targeted therapy, and well-coordinated and -funded domestic and international monitoring, tracking, and prevention and control plans) to respond to new drug-resistant threats. Finally, because it takes years to develop a new drug, planning must include consideration of needs that are immediate as well those that are anticipated to occur over the coming decade.

These concepts have been summarized succinctly and precisely by Nobel prize winner Dr. Joshua Lederberg, who stated, "The future of humanity and microbes will likely evolve as . . . episodes of our wits versus their genes."

Resistant Infections in Hospitals Kill 90,000 Each Year in the United States

Arthur Allen

Arthur Allen, a writer and journalist based in Washington D.C., is the author of the book, Vaccine: The Controversial Story of Medicine's Greatest Lifesaver *(2007).*

If you are an American admitted to a hospital in Amsterdam, Toronto, or Copenhagen these days, you'll be considered a biohazard. Doctors and nurses will likely put you into quarantine while they determine whether you're carrying methicillin-resistant Staphylococcus aureus, a deadly organism that is increasingly common stateside, especially in our hospitals. And if you test positive for methicillin-resistant staph, or MRSA, these European and Canadian hospital workers will don protective gloves, masks, and gowns each time they approach you, and then strip off the gear and scrub down vigorously when they leave your room. The process is known as "search and destroy"—a combat mission that hospitals abroad are undertaking to prevent the spread of germs that resist antibiotics. Our own health authorities, meanwhile, have been strangely reluctant to join the assault.

In the United States, MRSA kills an estimated 13,000 people every year, which means that a hospital patient is 10 times as likely to die of MRSA as an inmate is to be murdered in prison. The latest survey by the Centers for Disease Control and Prevention found that 64 percent of the Staphylococcus-aureus strains in American hospitals were MRSA—that is, resistant to the powerful antibiotic methicillin and other antibiotics—which makes them difficult to treat. MRSA has also spread to the general public, afflicting football teams and schools in the last three years. I know a healthy 5-year-old who got a staph infection recently after she skinned her knee on the playground. She ended up requiring two full months of antibiotic treatment, while her mother scoured the house with bleach on doctor's orders. And she may not be rid of the bug yet.

Given the dimensions of the threat, you'd think that the CDC would be making a priority of fighting it. After all, federal health agencies have spent billions to fight anthrax (which caused five deaths in 2001), smallpox (last U.S. death: 1949), and pandemic flu (yet to appear in the United States). And there is reason to think that search and destroy works, since health-care authorities abroad have kept rates of antibiotic-resistant bugs in their countries much lower than ours. In Dutch hospitals, the rate of MRSA is less than 1 percent. Canada's rate is 10 percent. And more than 100 studies have shown the effectiveness of search and destroy, including work released in the United States.

Yet the CDC refuses to endorse search and destroy. It is sticking to the mantra that hospital workers should wash their hands more carefully and frequently, and that in most cases patients should be isolated only after symptoms of infection with MRSA appear. Routine surveillance to find patients who may not be symptomatic, but are still contagious, is rarely practiced, and not recommended in the CDC's new hospital infection-fighting guidelines, which were released last week after five years of deliberations. The guidelines do not include a routine recommendation for search and destroy.

This is a bitter pill for infectious-disease experts, who have been joined by the relatives of dead patients, Consumers Union, and even a few Congress members in pressing the CDC. "Why are we spending millions if not billions on bird flu, a ghost that might not happen, when you have thousands being colonized by MRSA and dying of it?" asks Dr. William

Jarvis, a top CDC hospital-infection expert until he resigned in 2003. At a March 29 hearing on hospital infections—which, all told, kill an estimated 90,000 patients each year—Rep. Bart Stupak, D-Mich., charged that the CDC had stood by, despite a steady rise in infections since the early 1970s. "During that time, hospital stays have grown dramatically shorter yet infection rates continue to go up," Stupak said. "What do we have to do to motivate CDC?"

The CDC refuses to endorse search and destroy. It is sticking to the mantra that hospital workers should wash their hands more carefully and frequently.

Of course, many who succumb to hospital infections are already old, weak, and sick. And fighting such infections is a complicated, laborious business. Bacteria are everywhere, and each type of medical intervention, whether it be open-heart surgery, hip replacement, or traumatic wound care, carries specific risks of infection and methods for avoiding them. The Dutch approach is to test all high-risk patients before they are admitted. High risk, in practice, means diabetics, kidney-dialysis patients, and anyone who has been in a high-risk environment, such as a nursing home—or, from the point of view of the Dutch, the United States.

It's far more effective to isolate carriers, who may not yet be sick with the resistant microbes, than to wait until you have a confirmed infection, says Dr. Jan Kluytmans, a leading Dutch combatant in the resistance wars. Kluytmans' hospital in Breda, Netherlands, has had only one hospital-acquired MRSA infection since 2001, out of perhaps 40,000 patients. He estimates that the technique has prevented about 150 deaths. The University of Virginia Hospital in Charlottesville imposed the same system in 1980, and has maintained lower rates of MRSA than hospitals of comparable size. In late 2002, Rhode Island Hospital in Providence began search and destroy, and the MRSA infection rate at the hospital has dropped 43 percent, says chief epidemiologist Dr. Leonard Mermel, while it has continued to rise at most other hospitals in New England.

The biggest push for search and destroy may come, sadly, from the threat of lawsuits.

The counterargument is made by Dr. Robert Weinstein, a hospital-infection expert at Cook County Hospital in Chicago, and a leader on the CDC advisory committee that issued last week's guidelines. Weinstein argues that isolated patients generally get lousier care. And while aggressive action against MRSA may lower rates of that infection, he says, it doesn't necessarily reduce the incidence of deadly infections overall. Weinstein isn't against hospitals trying search and destroy. But he doesn't think it should become the standard of care until more studies prove its efficacy.

With a few exceptions, American hospitals, for their part, have been leery of the short-term expense and staff burden posed by search and destroy. A quick nasal swab of an admitted patient may cost only $20, but the nursing staff has to carefully monitor isolated patients, and find room to house them. The hospitals' reluctance may be shortsighted, however: A recent study shared that the average hospital infection adds $20,000 to a patient's bill. And while hospitals have traditionally passed on their costs to other payers, Medicare—which sets reimbursement standards—is starting to curtail payments to cover hospital errors, and may eventually stop paying to treat infections that could have been prevented.

The biggest push for search and destroy may come, sadly, from the threat of lawsuits. Several large ones have been settled with hospitals where patients died of infections. Fifteen states have passed laws that require hospitals to report infection rates, and another 28 are considering such legislation. An infectious-disease specialist I know offers a much simpler prescription: Whatever you do, he says, stay out of hospitals.

Resistant Infections Can Be Deadly Even Outside Health Care Facilities

Alison Young

Alison Young is a reporter for The Atlanta Journal-Constitution, *a daily newspaper published in Atlanta, Georgia.*

D arriel Fleming thought he had a spider bite.

As the boil swelled painfully on his stomach, the 28-year-old Marietta [Georgia] man went to a nearby emergency room. A doctor drained the wound and sent Fleming home with a prescription for antibiotics.

Three weeks later, Fleming was dead, killed last July [2007] by a drug-resistant form of staph bacteria called MRSA.

MRSA, or methicillin-resistant Staphylococcus aureus, for decades was an infection confined to hospitals and nursing homes. But MRSA strains are increasingly infecting people in the community, outside of health care settings.

In Georgia, more than 1,700 people have been hospitalized in the past three years with severe MRSA infections caught in the community, according to reports filed with the state health department. At least 62 have died—including several children with a deadly form of MRSA pneumonia.

Local and federal health officials are working to educate doctors and the public about the rise in these drug-resistant infections—best evaluated and treated early—and on ways people can protect themselves. They emphasize that the vast majority of community MRSA infections are treatable skin boils and abscesses.

Sometimes, for reasons unclear to scientists, the bacteria invade a person's bloodstream or wreak havoc with internal organs.

Researchers are studying who gets these serious community MRSA infections and examining the bacteria for clues about why they live on some people without causing infection—yet kill others.

About 85 percent of life-threatening, invasive MRSA infections involve people who have been hospitalized, lived in a nursing home or been treated in some other health care facility.

"We want people to understand that potentially, even though it's very uncommon, these community MRSA cases can be very serious and even fatal," said Dr. Rachel Gorwitz, epidemiologist at the Centers for Disease Control and Prevention [CDC, the nation's top health agency].

Community vs. Hospital MRSA

Staph bacteria, even those that aren't resistant to antibiotics, have long caused serious infections.

In the 1960s, the first reports surfaced of staph infections that had stopped responding to the antibiotic methicillin. Over the decades, those strains have spread, and the germs have developed resistance to other drugs, largely in hospitals where they infect patients weakened by disease or made vulnerable through surgical wounds and catheters.

Even today, MRSA poses the greatest threat in hospitals, where strains are usually genetically different and, because of antibiotic use, more difficult to kill than those circulating out in the community. About 85 percent of life-threatening, invasive MRSA infections involve people who have been hospitalized, lived in a nursing home or been treated in some other health care facility, the CDC estimates.

During the 1980s, doctors began finding cases of MRSA in people who hadn't spent time in health care settings.

Unlike hospital strains, MRSA in the community tended to cause skin infections—pus-filled pimples and boils.

[A 2007 study] estimated invasive MRSA infections—in both health care facilities and the community—killed nearly 19,000 Americans in 2005.

Unlike their hospital cousins, community MRSA still responds to a wider range of antibiotics, experts said. It's unusual for community infections to become life-threatening.

Panic and MRSA

Still, MRSA made headlines last fall [2007]—and caused the panicked closure of some schools in Georgia and across the nation—in the wake of publicity about a new study estimating that more life-threatening infections occur than previously thought.

The study, which involved CDC and Emory University researchers, estimated invasive MRSA infections—in both health care facilities and the community—killed nearly 19,000 Americans in 2005. Another 94,000 had life-threatening infections.

In Atlanta, the study said, the incidence of invasive MRSA has increased 71 percent in recent years—from 19.3 infections per 100,000 people in 2001–02 to 33 infections in 2005, the most recent data analyzed.

About the same time, news reports played up the MRSA death of a Virginia teen. As public awareness and concern grew, schools in Georgia and elsewhere sent home notes alerting parents when a child had a routine, treatable MRSA boil. Some schools closed for disinfection.

Lost in the furor was the study's main finding: Most life-threatening MRSA infections—85 percent—involve people who have been infected while hospitalized or living in a nursing home. Only about 15 percent happened in the community.

People 65 and older were most likely to suffer invasive MRSA infections of all types, the study found. Black people had invasive MRSA at nearly twice the rate of whites, which researchers speculate could be due to higher rates of chronic illnesses that may make them more vulnerable.

Contrary to public perception during last fall's [2007] panic, school-age children aren't at greatest risk for serious MRSA infections—nor is scrubbing surfaces an effective way of preventing transmission of bacteria spread by skin-to-skin contact or by sharing intimate items, such as towels, razors or sports equipment.

Awareness, Not Panic

Dr. Susan Ray, an associate professor of medicine at Emory and a co-author of the study, said the public needs to be aware that MRSA is in the community—but not become panicked by it.

"Most people who have a skin infection with staph germs have a boil that comes and goes and they may never have seen a doctor," Ray said.

Experts don't know why MRSA ravages some people and not others.

Those who seek help from a doctor usually are successfully treated.

Dr. Amy Kim, an Atlanta dermatologist, says she sees about one or two MRSA cases every week out of about 150 patients. Usually, the patients are in their 20s or 30s, and they're seeking treatment for boils, abscesses or inflamed pus-filled pimples around their hair follicles.

The diagnosis isn't what patients want to hear.

"People are pretty freaked out about it," Kim said. She tries to reassure them that, while MRSA is resistant to some antibiotics, it's still very treatable with others. Nearly all her patients' infections have cleared up within 10 days. In rare cases, however, the bacteria can enter the bloodstream—with deadly consequences. Being elderly, having skin problems or in poor health may be contributing factors for invasive infections.

Experts don't know why MRSA ravages some people and not others.

"That's the $64,000 question," said Ray. "We don't know."

Grief and Frustration

That such a young man like Darriel Fleming would die so suddenly left his wife reeling with grief and unanswered questions.

Although records show doctors reported Fleming's community-associated MRSA death to the state, his widow said she never knew the bacteria killed her husband until contacted by *The Atlanta Journal-Constitution* [*AJC*].

"I'm just so frustrated," said Cynthia Fleming. "I'm just trying to come to grips with this."

Hospital records, obtained by the *AJC* with Cynthia Fleming's authorization, show her husband's infection was caused by MRSA.

She wonders whether her husband could have been saved if he had been diagnosed earlier with MRSA.

Darriel Fleming, who had heart disease and was a diabetic at risk of skin problems, went to WellStar Cobb Hospital in Austell on June 17 [2007] after a painful boil grew on his stomach. In the emergency room, the doctor lanced the abscess and packed it with gauze.

The doctor didn't say what it was, said Cynthia Fleming, who went to the hospital with Darriel that day. "My husband kept saying it was a spider bite. I kept saying it doesn't look like a spider bite to me," she said.

Darriel Fleming was sent home with a prescription for Bactrim, an antibiotic, although no lab tests were done on the abscess to determine what organism caused it, hospital records show.

About three weeks later, on July 5, Fleming developed a fever of 104 degrees. The next day, he went back to the hospital. While a chest X-ray was ordered, again the hospital didn't run any blood tests to look for an infection, hospital and insurance records show. The hospital sent him home with instructions to take Tylenol and drink fluids.

Less than 24 hours later, Fleming was extremely ill and back at the emergency room. Despite being put on powerful, intravenous antibiotics, including vancomycin, Fleming's condition declined rapidly.

He was put on a ventilator in the hospital's intensive care unit, but died at 3:14 a.m. on July 8 [2007].

Final blood culture results, which came back after Fleming died, showed the Marietta man's bloodstream infection was caused by MRSA. A separate culture of his abdominal wound—taken less than an hour before he died—found MRSA there as well, hospital records show.

The tests indicated the MRSA bacteria infecting Fleming should have been susceptible to being killed by Bactrim, the antibiotic he was prescribed June 17. Why it didn't work may never be known.

Hospital officials refused to discuss Fleming's case, even with his widow's permission.

In general, emergency room doctors assume that abscesses involve MRSA, said Dr. Gerald Bortolazzo, chairman of ApolloMD, the firm that employs the hospital's ER doctors. Patients are given Bactrim, the preferred antibiotic for strains circulating in Atlanta.

Searching for Answers

At the CDC's campus on Clifton Road in Atlanta [Georgia], scientists in the national Staphylococcus reference laboratory examine samples of MRSA from people like Darriel Fleming.

They grow the bacteria in large incubators, then determine what antibiotics will and won't kill them. They also run tests to identify the bacteria's genetic fingerprints and whether they are producing certain toxins.

A lot remains unknown about MRSA—especially why it lives on some people without infecting them, and why in some cases it kills.

"That's really an important question for us to learn more about," said Gorwitz, the CDC epidemiologist.

It may involve differences within MRSA strains, a person's genetics or delays in seeking care, she said.

Until scientists have more answers, experts said, the public's best protection is to practice good hygiene and get skin problems checked out by a doctor.

U.S. Deaths from Staph Infections May Exceed the Number of Deaths from AIDS

The Associated Press

The Associated Press *is the largest news organization in the world, providing a source of news, photos, graphics, audio, and video for thousands of daily newspaper, radio, television, and online customers.*

More than 90,000 Americans get potentially deadly infections each year from a drug-resistant staph "superbug," the government reported Tuesday [October 16, 2007] in its first overall estimate of invasive disease caused by the germ.

Deaths tied to these infections may exceed those caused by AIDS, said one public health expert commenting on the new study. The report shows just how far one form of the staph germ has spread beyond its traditional hospital setting.

The overall incidence rate was about 32 invasive infections per 100,000 people. That's an "astounding" figure, said an editorial in [October 2007 in the] *Journal of the American Medical Association*, which published the study.

Most drug-resistant staph cases are mild skin infections. But this study focused on invasive infections—those that enter the bloodstream or destroy flesh and can turn deadly.

Carried by Healthy People

Researchers found that only about one-quarter involved hospitalized patients. However, more than half were in the health care system—people who had recently had surgery or were on

The Associated Press, "'Superbug' Deaths Could Surpass AIDS: Drug-Resistant Germs Becoming More Common, Government Report Finds," MSNBC.com, October 16, 2007. Republished with permission of MSNBC.com, conveyed through Copyright Clearance Center, Inc.

kidney dialysis, for example. Open wounds and exposure to medical equipment are major ways the bug spreads.

In recent years, the resistant germ has become more common in hospitals and it has been spreading through prisons, gyms and locker rooms, and in poor urban neighborhoods.

The new study offers the broadest look yet at the pervasiveness of the most severe infections caused by the bug, called methicillin-resistant Staphylococcus aureus, or MRSA. These bacteria can be carried by healthy people, living on their skin or in their noses.

In recent years, the resistant [staph] germ has . . . been spreading through prisons, gyms and locker rooms, and in poor urban neighborhoods.

An invasive form of the disease is being blamed for the death Monday [October 15, 2007] of a 17-year-old Virginia high school senior. Doctors said the germ had spread to his kidneys, liver, lungs and muscles around his heart.

The researchers' estimates are extrapolated from 2005 surveillance data from nine mostly urban regions considered representative of the country. There were 5,287 invasive infections reported that year in people living in those regions, which would translate to an estimated 94,360 cases nationally, the researchers said.

Most cases were life-threatening bloodstream infections. However, about 10 percent involved so-called flesh-eating disease, according to the study led by researchers at the federal Centers for Disease Control and Prevention (CDC).

There were 988 reported deaths among infected people in the study, for a rate of 6.3 per 100,000. That would translate to 18,650 deaths annually, although the researchers don't know if MRSA was the cause in all cases.

Curb Antibiotic Use

If these deaths all were related to staph infections, the total would exceed other better-known causes of death including AIDS—which killed an estimated 17,011 Americans in 2005—said Dr. Elizabeth Bancroft of the Los Angeles County Health Department, the editorial author.

The results underscore the need for better prevention measures. That includes curbing the overuse of antibiotics and improving hand-washing and other hygiene procedures among hospital workers, said the CDC's Dr. Scott Fridkin, a study co-author.

Some hospitals have drastically cut infections by first isolating new patients until they are screened for MRSA.

The bacteria don't respond to penicillin-related antibiotics once commonly used to treat them, partly because of overuse. They can be treated with other drugs but health officials worry that their overuse could cause the germ to become resistant to those, too.

A survey earlier this year [2007] suggested that MRSA infections, including noninvasive mild forms, affect 46 out of every 1,000 U.S. hospital and nursing home patients—or as many as 5 percent. These patients are vulnerable because of open wounds and invasive medical equipment that can help the germ spread.

Dr. Buddy Creech, an infectious disease specialist at Vanderbilt University, said the *JAMA* [*Journal of the American Medical Association*] study emphasizes the broad scope of the drug-resistant staph "epidemic," and highlights the need for a vaccine, which he called "the holy grail of staphylococcal research."

The regions studied were: the Atlanta metropolitan area; Baltimore, Md.; the state of Connecticut; Davidson County, Tenn.; the Denver metropolitan area; Monroe County, NY; the Portland, Ore. metropolitan area; Ramsey County, Minn.; and the San Francisco metropolitan area.

Drug-Resistant Staph Infections Are on the Rise in American Schools

Natasha Lindstrom

Natasha Lindstrom is a staff writer for the Daily Press, *a newspaper published in Victorville, California.*

A potentially fatal infection may be spreading to more students than ever before, but few school and county officials are tracking it.

Sometimes called the "superbug," methicillin-resistant Staphylococcus aureus, or MRSA, is a drug-resistant strain of staph infections that can be deadly if left untreated.

While concerns about the blood-borne bacterial infection were once relegated to hospitals or the occasional locker room, reports of the infections continue to rise in schools across the country.

MRSA Infections in Hesperia, California

"We've been seeing what we call the community-acquired strain of MRSA since 2001," said Registered Nurse Sean O'Grady, who works in the St. Mary Medical Center infection control department [in California] and has been educating local schools about the infections. "It has slowly been growing and growing, and now it's worldwide."

The MRSA infection, which typically manifests as pimples and boils, does not respond to penicillin or related antibiotics, though it can be treated with other drugs. The infection can turn deadly if it enters the bloodstream or morphs into a flesh-eating wound.

Natasha Lindstrom, "Drug-Resistant Staph Infections on the Rise in Schools," *Daily Press* (Victorville, CA), October 8, 2008. Reproduced by permission.

"There isn't a school that hasn't been touched by MRSA," said Peggy Lindsay, school nurse for the Hesperia Unified School District [in California].

Four years ago, Hesperia's school district recorded only 12 infections, all of which affected athletes or a coach, Lindsay said.

But last year staph infections in Hesperia's school district topped three digits, with 120 cases—about two-thirds of which were MRSA, Lindsay said.

At least 24 students have contracted staph infections in the Hesperia district since the school year began eight weeks ago [August 2008], Lindsay said. No students have been seriously injured, but about half of those cases were MRSA, she said.

Next week [October 2008] the Hesperia district will hand deliver a "Parent's Guide to MRSA" to every student. Lindsay said parents have no reason to panic, but should encourage good hygiene and know how to spot an infection.

The Victor Valley Union High School District [VVUHSD] does not track staph infections at local schools, although Superintendent Julian Weaver said he would be open to having district-level discussions about tracking the cases.

"I would love to see us keeping track of that," said Janie Rehrer, the VVUHSD district nurse.

At least one of the district's schools—Victor Valley High School—had five students contract staph infections last year [2007], said athletic trainer Bridget Cummins.

The chance of a child becoming seriously ill or dying from a staph infection may be rare—but it does happen.

The Apple Valley Unified School District has not heard of any staph infections this year or last year, but also does not require schools to report the cases, according to the district office.

After two days of phone calls, officials at the Victor Elementary and Adelanto school districts could not be reached for comment.

Countywide, cases of staph infections are nearly impossible to track, as neither the San Bernardino County Superintendent of Schools nor the San Bernardino County Department of Public Health identify staph infections as a "reportable disease."

This is the first year the county health department does require hospitals to report staph aureus infections, but only those that cause a person to be hospitalized in intensive care or result in death, said Lea Morgan, public health program coordinator in the county's disease control section. The county has recorded 22 such cases since February [2008].

Staph Infections Can Be Deadly

The chance of a child becoming seriously ill or dying from a staph infection may be rare—but it does happen.

Last week [October 2008], an 18-year-old football player died from a methicillin-resistant Staphylococcus aureus infection in Kissimme, Fla., and on Sept. 2, a 14-year-old girl died from a staph infection in Winchester, Ky., according to *Associated Press* reports.

"The immune system of a child is not as robust as an adult's, and the longer it goes without treatment, the more risk you have of it being more severe," said Dr. James Kyle, vice president of medical affairs at St. Mary Medical Center.

As many as 90,000 people contract a staph infection in the United States each year, according to a study by the Centers for Disease Control and Prevention.

The study found nearly 19,000 died from staph infections in 2005—higher than the number of people who die in the United States each year from AIDS.

The infection is spread through skin-to-skin contact with an infected person or by touching surfaces that someone else has infected, such as towels, athletic equipment or tabletops.

While no local students have seriously suffered from the infections, it's important to check for red, hard skin or open sores, often mistaken for a spider bite that won't heal, said Peggy Lindsay, school nurse for the Hesperia Unified School District.

Resistant Infections Could Be a Huge Problem in the Event of a Pandemic

Anthony L. Kimery

Anthony L. Kimery, a journalist who has covered national and global security, intelligence, and defense issues for two decades, is online editor/senior reporter and editor of Homeland Security Insight and Analysis, *an electronic newsletter.*

Pandemic health preparedness authorities, virologists, and other scientists are expressing alarm over the findings of two new studies that indicate a potentially significant number of people died during the horrific 1918 influenza pandemic in part because highly opportunistic bacterial infections were able to flourish in these flu victims because the virus severely weakened their immune systems.

Scientists today also have found that the virulent H5N1 flu virus profoundly short circuits a person's immune system, especially people with healthy systems.

But what's of particularly grave concern is that a terribly weakened immune system is vulnerable to aggressive bacterial infections like the virulent strain of *Staphylococcus aureus* that's been linked to seasonal influenza deaths and has developed a resistance to many of the antibiotics used to treat it.

The Findings

Last fall [2007], the *Journal of the American Medical Association (JAMA)* reported that a strain of methicillin-resistant *Staphylococcus aureus* (MRSA) that has been spreading across the country is causing more life-threatening infections than public health authorities had thought, and killing more people in the US each year than AIDS.

Anthony L. Kimery, "Antibiotic Resistant Infections Will Be Problem During Pandemic," *Homeland Security Today*, August 19, 2008. Reproduced by permission.

The revelation that a pandemic strain of influenza could hasten the spread of antibiotic resistant bacterial infections like MRSA in flu patients is especially disturbing, and presents an entirely new set of challenges for pandemic preparedness planners.

HSToday.us [a Web site that discusses topics related to homeland security] earlier reported that hospital-acquired infections (HAIs) like MRSA that kill an estimated 90,000 to 100,000 Americans each year during routine hospital stays could be expected to run rampant during a health crisis in which tens of thousands—or more—persons require emergency medical care under what will likely be less than sterile and sanitary conditions. Conditions most authorities agree are primarily responsible for the transmission of HAIs like MRSA.

HAI infections can cause serious illnesses and, in severe cases, death. Indeed, infectious diseases are a major cause of illness, disability and death, statistics and authorities point out.

A pandemic strain of influenza could hasten the spread of antibiotic resistant bacterial infections . . . in flu patients.

The Need for Both Antivirals and Antibiotics

Consequently, "we have to realize that it isn't just antivirals that we need" during a pandemic, said Dr. Anthony Fauci, director of the National Institute of Allergy and Infectious Diseases and coauthor of one of the studies published in the *Journal of Infectious Diseases.*

"We need to make sure that we're prepared to treat people with antibiotics," Fauci stressed.

"Yes, of course bacterial infection following influenza should be of concern, and antibiotic resistant bacteria of even greater concern," Dr. Graeme Laver told *HSToday.us.*

A former professor of biochemistry and molecular biology at the John Curtin School of Medical Research at the Australian National University in Canberra, Laver played a key role in the development of the antivirals Tamiflu and Relenza.

Laver has been studying influenza viruses for nearly 40 years. Along with colleague Dr. Robert Webster, the two are credited with having first found the link between human flu and bird flu. In the 1960s, both received world acclaim when they developed a new and innovative generation of vaccines for flu viruses.

Preventing Severe Immune Reactions

Both new studies—the other published in *Emerging Infectious Diseases*—indicate that opportunistic infections are able to take hold in the upper respiratory tract of flu victims because of the flu's ability to provoke a severe immune system reaction called a "cytokine storm."

This problem is prevalent in victims infected with the H5N1 flu virus which, unlike seasonal flu viruses, upsets the chemical messengers that regulate immune function in a healthy, vigorous immune system, thus activating an inordinate number of immune cells.

Studies show children and teens between birth and 19 years of age account for nearly 46 percent of all H5N1 flu deaths in the world.

Similarly, the 1918 pandemic flu virus struck down an inordinate number of young, healthy adults.

Prior to the new studies linking virulent influenza to the onset of opportunistic bacterial infections, a team led by Menno de Jong of the Oxford University Clinical Research Unit in Ho Chi Minh City, Vietnam, urged that "the focus of clinical [pandemic] management should be on preventing this intense cytokine response by early diagnosis and effective antiviral treatment."

"If virus replication can be stopped in the early stages, then the likelihood of bacterial infection will be greatly reduced," Laver said.

Laver earlier explained to *HSToday.us* that "If people with flu symptoms take Tamiflu immediately, say within six or so hours after symptom onset, the infection should be rapidly terminated, the person should recover, and then, and this is important, should then be immune to reinfection for the rest of the pandemic."

Laver said "this has been called 'Aborted-infection Immunization,' and to use Tamiflu in this way would allow many health care workers and so on to go about their business without fear of reinfection."

Animals Also Are at Risk of Developing Resistant Infections

Christie Keith

Christie Keith is a contributing editor for Pet Connection, *a weekly pet care feature syndicated to newspapers, magazines, and Web sites in the United States and Canada.*

There's a new and growing threat to your pets' health, and while I wish I could tell you it's just another Internet rumor, it's all too real. I should know, because my dog is its latest poster child. I'm talking about something you might have thought only affected humans: drug-resistant staph infections.

We hear a lot about these types of infections in people these days, severe ones spread in hospitals and less severe ones spread in daycare centers, schools and gyms. Most human infections involve methicillin-resistant *Staphylococcus aureus*, or MRSA. In dogs and cats, the bacteria is slightly different—methicillin-resistant *staphylococcus intermedius*, or MRSI—but it's otherwise pretty much the same problem: some strains of a common bacteria found in and on most dogs, people and surfaces have evolved to resist the antibiotics we normally use to treat it.

Kyrie and Angelina's Battle with MRSI

My introduction to MRSI began three months ago, when I noticed my 9-year-old borzoi, Kyrie, had a small, quarter-sized red patch on her hip that seemed to hurt her terribly. I got her into the vet the next day, and she diagnosed a spider bite, shaved and cleaned the area, and put her on antibiotics, pain medication and a topical lidocaine spray to numb the wound. She predicted Kyrie would feel better in around 48 hours.

But Kyrie spent the night restless and whimpering despite the pain medication. And the next day, her coin-sized sore had become 8-by-8 inches of infected, oozing, red, raw skin. Unable to sleep while she was so uncomfortable, I spent a few hours on the Internet, where I learned two things. One, there are no venomous spiders in San Francisco, where we live, and two, most diagnosed spider bites are really something else entirely: drug resistant staph infections.

I took Kyrie to a specialist in the morning, and she agreed that her sore was almost certainly caused by MRSI. She put her on a different, hopefully more effective antibiotic while we waited for the results of a skin culture test which would determine what kinds of bacteria were present and what antibiotics would be effective.

At the same time Kyrie's infection was diagnosed, San Diego's Mary Ann Rose was trying to figure out why her Scottish Deerhound, Angelina, was not recovering from surgery for injuries received when she was hit by a car two weeks earlier. Rose and her husband are both physicians and Angelina had the best possible care at every stage. And yet, while she did fairly well when taking a 10-day course of prescribed post-surgery antibiotics, she went rapidly downhill in the 48 hours after the antibiotic treatment was done.

"She became very ill," Rose said. "She was weak, wouldn't eat, and had a fever for the first time since the accident." Over the next few hours, Angelina developed multiple ulcerated skin lesions all over her body.

Rose didn't waste any time. "I took her back in to the surgery clinic where she was operated on. It was a Saturday. They took one look at her and called board certified veterinary dermatologist Laura Stokking and said, 'We don't know what this is, but this is a really sick dog.' Dr. Stokking worked on her all day. She had IVs, and every inch of her body was cultured."

While caring for Angelina that day, Stokking saw evidence of some type of staphylococcus under the microscope. Knowing the dog had already been on two antibiotics that normally kill that bug, she started her on a different oral antibiotic as well as an anti-bacterial skin wash while awaiting test results. Angelina improved on the new treatment, and when the culture results came back, they confirmed that she had MRSI.

My dog Kyrie's culture showed she had MRSI as well. In fact, it indicated that two organisms were present. One was just what we expected, a methicillin-resistant staph, sensitive to a number of drugs including the one she was taking. But the other was a multi-drug resistant staph that was sensitive to almost none of the common veterinary antibiotics.

Still, Kyrie had gotten better while on the drug, so we continued the treatment and hoped for the best. Unfortunately, after the three-week course was finished, her symptoms returned with a vengeance. Back to the vet, where we faced some bad news about our options: amikacin, a drug that needs to be given intravenously every day, costs in the four figures, and has some very dangerous side effects; or chloramphenicol, a drug that wasn't included in the skin culture test that might or might not be effective.

I decided to go with the second option, primarily to avoid the stress of daily vet visits for Kyrie, and because the side effect risk, although far from negligible, was less for chloramphenicol. And at first, I assumed we'd gotten lucky, because the wound started healing immediately.

Unfortunately, it came back two days after a three-week course of chloramphenicol was finished, just like before. But I'd spent those three weeks researching MRSI and MRSA skin infections, and this time I tried dressings of medical-grade honey, which is often effective when used in combination with oral antibiotics. Within a few hours, the wound had started healing, and within two days it was finally gone. Today, three months after it all began, the infection seems to be eradicated, her coat has re-grown in the affected area, and we're hoping her next skin culture will show her to be free of the super-bugs.

Meanwhile, down in San Diego, Angelina was fighting for her life. "She had an episode of septicemia (blood infection), and the sores were all over her body, and the hair just sloughed off, and they were oozing," said Rose. "I have never seen a dog that sick that survived."

The Roses and their veterinarians persisted with Angelina's treatment, and gradually she recovered. After just under a month, they tried to stop the antibiotic, but her symptoms returned almost immediately.

In the end, Angelina was on the drug for more than 12 weeks before her cultures came back negative for MRSI. "She's lost most of her hair," said Rose. "My husband, who is an infectious disease doctor, says that in humans, when you get these resistant staphylococcus infections, they will slough skin for several months." In addition to the lingering skin and coat problems, Angelina suffered damage that will probably be permanent to the joints in one of her legs that had become infected.

There's no question the [MRSI] infections ... are becoming more widespread [in pets].

I spoke with Angelina's veterinary dermatologist, Laura Stokking, and she said that, while Angelina's case was a bad one, she's seen worse. "You know, it was easy with Angelina's parents because they're physicians, so they know a lot more," she said. "She responded pretty well. I have some cases where there is a substantially higher amount of the body that's affected and a lot more tissue necrosis, and the dogs are really systemically ill." She attributed Angelina's recovery, slow though it's been, to aggressive treatment.

MRSI on the Rise

I asked Stokking if it's just a coincidence that I heard of two cases at the same time, or if MRSI in pets is really on the rise. She said that MRSI infections were the hottest topic at the recent North American Veterinary Dermatology Forum, and while there is some increased awareness leading to more frequent diagnosis, there's no question the infections themselves are becoming more widespread.

The origin of most MRSI infections in pets is unclear.

"Definitely in dogs it's an emerging problem," she told me. "Up until recently, the bacteria that most commonly affected dogs didn't tend to trade resistance information with other bacteria the same way that the staph in humans did." Those days are gone, however, and she says both the incidence and prevalence of drug resistant bacteria are spreading in companion animals.

Given that MRSI infections are of increasing risk to dogs and cats, the most useful information a pet owner could get would be how to prevent them. To do that however, we'd need to know where the pets were getting the infections.

While humans frequently get the more severe strains of MRSA in hospitals, Kyrie was perfectly healthy and hadn't even been to the vet's office recently. And even though Angelina had recently undergone surgery and spent time in a veterinary hospital, she actually had the infection, although it was undiagnosed, prior to her accident and surgery, in the form of two lumps on her legs—lumps that were initially mistaken for spider bites.

Stokking agreed that the origin of most MRSI infections in pets is unclear, and wasn't surprised that Angelina most likely had acquired the bacteria before her surgery. "We don't usually see a link between hospitalization or veterinary visits and the acquisition of this strain of staphylococcus," she said.

What about the canine or feline equivalents of the daycare center or gym, such as dog parks, boarding kennels or groomers? "Contaminated water, contaminated shampoo bottles," she agreed. "It's possible."

Pets living in the same household with an infected dog or cat will sometimes get MRSI from the sick pet. (Humans virtually never get MRSI from animals, although we can transmit MRSA to them.) But neither Rose's nor my other dogs became infected, and that's not uncommon. Why did seemingly healthy dogs like Kyrie and Angelina become ill, when other also seemingly healthy pets in the same household didn't?

The truth is, we really don't know where dogs and cats are being exposed to these bugs, which makes it almost impossible to prevent our pets from getting them.

However, uncertainty about prevention doesn't mean there's nothing pet owners can do to minimize their pets' risk of resistant infections. Because rapid diagnosis and effective treatment are key to preventing the more serious forms of the disease, pet owners and their veterinarians need to be on the lookout for it.

They first need to be aware that many skin infections with MRSI or MRSA are initially misdiagnosed as spider bites, as both Kyrie's and Angelina's were. Stokking said that the Centers for Disease Control and Prevention [CDC] have a poster used in human medicine that says, "Looks like a spider bite but isn't? MRSA." Since it's such a common misdiagnosis, she believes it's probably a good idea to do a skin culture on any suspected spider bite and any skin infection that doesn't immediately respond to the usual antibiotics.

Even though it was not the case for Kyrie or Angelina, there is one other factor that should make owners and veterinarians particularly alert for signs of MRSI in pets. "We do frequently see a history (in infected pets) of repeated use of antibiotics," Stokking told me.

Skin Cultures Are Important

Owners also need to be aware that trying to save money by delaying or skipping diagnostic tests can cost them much more money in the long run. A skin culture might cost over $100, but wasting time on an ineffective antibiotic can cost much more. The first drug Kyrie went on was priced at only around $40, but the second one was nearly 10 times that for a three-week supply.

And if you think my dog's prescription was expensive, want to know how much that course of amikacin—or, for that matter, vancomycin, the drug of last resort for resistant staph in humans—would cost? Around $1,000. Not to mention both have to be given intravenously and are highly toxic to the kidneys. Worse, over-reliance on vancomycin in human as well as veterinary medicine is leading to the further development of vancomycin-resistant bacteria, which is leading directly to the loss of human lives.

But the really bad news has nothing to do with your bank account. It has to do with the development of resistant bugs itself. Bacteria have a dazzling ability to trade genes and develop resistance, so strains that are susceptible to one drug today could easily be resistant to it tomorrow. Using an ineffective antibiotic, chosen without doing a skin culture first, can accelerate the development of additional resistance in bacteria. And that, again, threatens not only our pets but *human* health.

Given that risk and expense, as well as how painful and dangerous these infections are, an ounce of detection in the form of a culture may well be worth a pound of a very expensive cure.

"Don't be afraid to culture," Stokking said. "It's better to do a culture and then find out that it would have responded to cephalexin than not culture and let it go three weeks before realizing that you're dealing with a methicillin-resistant strain."

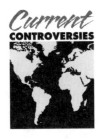

CHAPTER 2

Are Drug-Resistant Infections the Result of Agricultural Use of Antibiotics?

Chapter Preface

The discovery of penicillin—the world's first antibiotic drug—in 1928 by Scottish scientist Alexander Fleming revolutionized the treatment of infectious diseases. Bacterial illnesses often fatal in the past suddenly became easily curable, and the number of deaths caused by these pathogens dropped around the world. Since 1928, drug companies have developed more than a hundred different antibiotics used by today's doctors to treat a wide range of bacteria-related illnesses—everything from common childhood ear infections and minor skin infections to much more serious and potentially lethal infections such as meningitis. In recent decades, however, the widespread use of antibiotics has allowed many types of bacteria to develop a resistance to commonly used antibiotics, and many traditional antibiotic drugs have already lost much of their effectiveness.

One area of overuse is the prescription of antibiotics by doctors and hospitals. For years, doctors have prescribed antibiotics not only for serious diseases known to be bacterial in nature, but also for children and adults with upper respiratory infections, sinus infections, and ear infections—illnesses usually caused by viruses, not bacteria. This frequent use of antibiotics for viral health conditions, many commentators argue, has encouraged bacteria to develop resistance to many of the once-powerful antibiotic drugs in doctors' arsenals, and has led to a major public health crisis of resistant infections. Some antibiotic-resistant infections, such as methicillin-resistant *Staphylococcus aureus* (MRSA) are causing tens of thousands of deaths each year.

Doctors are tempted to prescribe antibiotics for several reasons. For example, in many cases, doctors cannot be sure of the cause of minor respiratory or other conditions without lab tests that could take several days. In an effort to treat patients quickly, many doctors decline to order testing and simply err on the side of prescribing antibiotics just in case the source is bacterial. Patients also place great pressure on doctors to prescribe antibiotics. The public has come to believe that antibiotics are wonder drugs, and many people do not understand the scientific distinction between viruses and bacteria. Experts also suggest another reason for the excessive reliance on antibiotics by doctors—drug companies that manufacture antibiotics have long promoted their products by offering literature, seminars, and in some cases, free drugs to doctors' offices. Although many doctors say they are not influenced by these sales pitches, these marketing efforts clearly help to familiarize doctors with antibiotic products and make it more likely that they will be prescribed.

The problem of over-prescription is compounded when patients fail to take the prescribed course of antibiotics. Typically, antibiotics must be taken consistently for periods ranging from five days to two weeks, and if the patient starts feeling better and stops taking the medication, not all the bacteria in the body will be killed. The bacteria that survive become stronger and multiply. If this happens repeatedly, some bacteria become resistant to that particular medicine, and eventually the antibiotic will fail to kill that type of bacteria. In the meantime, the antibiotic often kills good bacteria in the body, weakening the immune system and making it easier for the more resistant bacteria to create infection. Adding to the problem, patients often flush left-over antibiotic medications down the toilet, allowing them to become proliferate in the environment. Some health experts are concerned that this, too, has contributed to the problem of antibiotic resistance.

In hospitals, a similar scenario has been reported in which doctors prescribe the most powerful antibiotic available while awaiting lab tests to identify the particular type of bacteria that is afflicting the patient. Once the lab results are reported, however, many doctors fail to scale back to less powerful antibiotics that also could cure the patient. This overuse of newer, more powerful antibiotics helps bacteria to develop resistance more quickly than necessary to even the best antibiotics. Although this pattern of behavior may help individual patients, it adds to the public health problem of increasing bacterial resistance.

Individuals can help prevent this spiral of antibiotic resistance. First, patients should not demand antibiotics from their doctors and should take them only if really needed. Antibiotics should never be taken for common colds or flu, because these are always viral illnesses. If prescribed antibiotics, patients should take care to complete the course of antibiotics as directed, to kill the bacteria completely. People should never self-prescribe or take antibiotics prescribed to someone else or for an earlier illness, because antibiotics should be carefully prescribed to treat specific types of bacteria, which can vary for different types of infections. And patients should dispose of any left-over medication in the trash.

The overuse of antibiotics, however, is not confined to doctors and the medical field. Antibiotics are routinely used— even more so than they are used in human medicine—in agriculture to prevent illness in food animals such as chickens, pigs, and cattle. This chapter focuses on the problem of agricultural antibiotic use.

Seventy Percent of Antibiotic Drugs Are Used in Agriculture

Keep Antibiotics Working

Keep Antibiotics Working *is a coalition of concerned health, consumer, agricultural, environmental, humane and other advocacy groups that works to reduce the growing public health threat of antibiotic resistance by advocating for the reduction of antibiotics in animal agriculture.*

When bacteria are exposed to antibiotics, the bacteria resistant to these drugs live to reproduce. Thus, while antibiotics are important for disease treatment, their use creates stronger, more-resistant strains of bacteria over time. For this reason, it is important to use antibiotics only when it is absolutely necessary. Still, overuse of antibiotics occurs in both human medicine and animal agriculture.

Overuse of Antibiotics

Overuse in human medicine: Inappropriate prescriptions can elicit antibiotic-resistant bacteria. Patients often request—and doctors prescribe—antibiotics for viral infections such as the common cold, even though antibiotics cannot kill viruses. Failure of patients to complete prescriptions also promotes the survival of antibiotic-resistant bacteria.

The nontherapeutic use of antibiotics involves low-level exposure in feed over long periods—an ideal way to encourage bacteria to develop resistance.

Overuse in animal agriculture: While overuse in human medicine is a major part of the problem of antibiotic resistance, meat producers use an estimated 70 percent of all U.S.

Keep Antibiotics Working, "Factsheet: Antibiotic Resistance and Animal Agriculture," KeepAntibioticsWorking.com, 2004. Reproduced by permission.

antibiotics and related drugs nontherapeutically (i.e., as a routine feed additive to promote slightly faster growth and to compensate for unsanitary and crowded conditions). The amount of antibiotics used nontherapeutically in animal agriculture is eight times greater than the amount used in all of human medicine.

Furthermore . . .

- Many of the antibiotics used in animal agriculture are also used in human medicine.

- The nontherapeutic use of antibiotics involves low-level exposure in feed over long periods—an ideal way to encourage bacteria to develop resistance.

- A 2002 analysis of more than 500 scientific articles by the Alliance for the Prudent Use of Antibiotics (APUA), published in the peer-reviewed journal *Clinical Infectious Diseases*, found that "[m]any lines of evidence link antimicrobial-resistant human infections to foodborne pathogens of animal origin." The APUA report concluded that "the elimination of nontherapeutic use of antimicrobials in food animals . . . will lower the burden of antimicrobial resistance in the environment, with consequent benefits to human and animal health."

- Antibiotic-resistant bacteria can easily transfer their resistance traits to unrelated bacteria once inside the human body. Thus, development of resistance in all types of bacteria is of concern, regardless of whether those bacteria themselves cause disease.

- Resistant human diseases strongly linked to the agricultural overuse of antibiotics include food poisoning caused by *Salmonella* or *Campylobacter* and post-surgical infections caused by *Enterococcus*. A recent study has suggested a link between resistant urinary tract infections caused by *Escherichia coli* and food sources.

Resistant bacteria can be transferred from animals to humans in three ways:

Via food: Meat in grocery stores is widely contaminated with antibiotic-resistant bacteria. A study in the Washington, DC, area found 20 percent of the sampled meat was contaminated with *Salmonella* and 84 percent of those bacteria were resistant to antibiotics used in human medicine and animal agriculture.

Via working with animals: Workers in the livestock industry may pick up resistant bacteria by handling animals, feed, and manure. They can then transfer the bacteria to family and community members.

Via the environment: Groundwater, surface water, and soil are contaminated from the nearly two trillion pounds of manure generated in the United States each year. This manure contains resistant bacteria, creating an immense pool of resistance genes available for transfer to bacteria that cause human disease.

Reducing Antibiotic Overuse

The Centers for Disease Control [CDC, the nation's top health agency] is implementing extensive programs to educate both patients and physicians about reducing antibiotic overuse.

As noted in a 2003 National Academy of Sciences report, "[a] decrease in antimicrobial use in human medicine alone will have little effect on the current situation. Substantial efforts must be made to decrease inappropriate overuse in animals and agriculture as well."

Major reductions in animal use can be achieved by canceling existing approvals of medically important antibiotics for nontherapeutic purposes. Existing approvals can be cancelled by Congress through legislation or by the Food and Drug Administration (FDA) through regulation.

Although FDA acknowledges that antibiotic resistance is a problem, the agency is unable to cancel existing approvals within a reasonable time.

Congress must pass new legislation to curb antibiotic resistance because FDA cannot solve this problem in a reasonable time.

FDA can theoretically cancel drug approvals, yet prior cancellations have taken up to 20 years to complete per drug class. Seven important classes of antibiotics are currently used both in human medicine and as non-therapeutic feed additives.

Existing feed-additive approvals were issued decades ago; at that time, resistance was not a prominent public health issue and FDA did not subject drugs to detailed evaluations that considered antibiotic resistance.

In 2003, FDA released Guidance #152 acknowledging that use of antibiotics in animal agriculture is "a contributing factor to the development of [antibiotic] resistance."

FDA guidance strengthens the review of antibiotics that are proposed to be marketed in the future, but does not establish any schedule for reviewing or taking action on antibiotics already on the market.

Farmers practicing sustainable agriculture in the United States are already producing premium pork and chicken without antibiotics.

Congress must pass new legislation to curb antibiotic resistance because FDA cannot solve this problem in a reasonable time.

Real World Success Stories: Examples of Antibiotic Reduction

Large companies such as McDonald's and Bon Appétit have already taken steps to reduce antibiotic use in animal agriculture by their producers.

In 1998, Denmark—the world's largest pork exporter—enacted a ban on antibiotic feed additives. Producers adjusted to this ban by improving hygiene and animal husbandry standards. A study by the World Health Organization [WHO] concluded that Denmark reduced overall use of antibiotics in agriculture by 54 percent and experienced a "dramatic" reduction in resistant bacteria in animals, without causing consumer price increases or undermining animal health or food safety. A similar ban is now in force in all EU [European Union] countries.

Farmers practicing sustainable agriculture in the United States are already producing premium pork and chicken without antibiotics.

Transmission of Resistant Bacteria from Agriculture May Be Greater Than That from Hospitals

David L. Smith, Jonathan Dushoff, and J. Glenn Morris

David L. Smith is a mathematical epidemiologist and infectious disease ecologist at Fogarty International Center, National Institutes of Health, in Bethesda, Maryland. Jonathan Dushoff is on the research staff in the Department of Ecology and Evolutionary Biology at Princeton University. J. Glenn Morris, a physician epidemiologist and specialist in infectious diseases, is chair of the Department of Epidemiology and Preventive Medicine at the University of Maryland School of Medicine in Baltimore.

Like SARS [severe acute respiratory syndrome], Ebola, and other emerging infectious diseases, antibiotic resistance in bacteria may have a zoonotic origin [that is, transmitted from animals to humans]. Evidence suggests that antibiotic use in agriculture has contributed to antibiotic resistance in the pathogenic bacteria of humans, but the chain from cause to effect is long and complicated.

From Animals to Humans

Antibiotic use clearly selects for antibiotic resistance, but how far do these effects extend beyond the population where antibiotics are used? Antibiotics and antibiotic-resistant bacteria (ARB) are found in the air and soil around farms, in surface and ground water, in wild animal populations, and on retail meat and poultry. ARB are carried into the kitchen on contaminated meat and poultry, where other foods are cross-

David L. Smith, Jonathan Dushoff, and J. Glenn Morris, "Agricultural Antibiotics and Human Health: Does Antibiotic Use in Agriculture Have a Greater Impact Than Hospital Use?" *PLoS Medicine*, July 5, 2005. Reproduced by Permission.

contaminated because of common unsafe handling practices. Following ingestion, bacteria occasionally survive the formidable but imperfect gastric barrier, and colonize the gut.

The impact of agricultural antibiotic use remains controversial and poorly quantified.

Patterns of colonization (asymptomatic carriage) and infection (symptomatic carriage) in human populations provide additional evidence that ARB occasionally move from animals to humans. The strongest evidence comes from the history of the use of antibiotics for growth promotion in Europe. After first Denmark and then the European Union [EU] banned the use of antibiotics for growth promotion, prevalence of resistant bacteria declined in farm animals, in retail meat and poultry, and within the general human population.

Despite the evidence linking bacterial antibiotic resistance on farms to resistance in humans, the impact of agricultural antibiotic use remains controversial and poorly quantified. This is partly because of the complex of population-level processes underlying the between-species ("heterospecific") and within-species, host-to-host ("horizontal") spread of ARB. To emerge as human pathogens, new strains of ARB must (1) evolve, originating from mutations or gene transfer; (2) spread, usually horizontally among humans or animals, but occasionally heterospecifically; and (3) cause disease.

All three of these steps are complex and imperfectly understood. The emergence of a new type of resistance is a highly random event, which can't be predicted accurately, and may involve multiple steps that preclude perfect understanding even after the fact. Spread is equally complicated and may obscure the origins of resistance. In some cases, emergence of resistance in one bacterial species is a consequence of the emergence and spread in another species, followed by the transfer of resistance genes from one bacterial species to another. Because of the underlying complexity, mathematical models are necessary to develop theory—a qualitative understanding of the underlying epidemiological processes. Theory helps researchers organize facts, identify missing information, design surveillance, and analyze data.

Horizontal Transmission

Theory clearly shows that the impact of agricultural antibiotic use depends on whether resistant bacteria have high, low, or intermediate horizontal transmission rates in human populations. The rate of horizontal transmission among humans is determined by the underlying biology of the pathogen, medical antibiotic use, and hospital infection control, but not by agricultural antibiotic use. On the other hand, a farm where multiple antibiotics are used routinely, universally, and in low quantities for growth promotion is likely to be an excellent environment for the evolution of multiple resistance factors, including some variants that might never have evolved in humans. Thus, even very rare transmission resulting from agricultural antibiotics may have a medical impact by introducing new resistant variants to the human population. The epidemiology of spread in the human population dictates how the impact of agricultural antibiotic use should be assessed.

Zoonotic pathogens, such as *Campylobacter* and *Salmonella,* are generally regarded as having low horizontal transmission rates in human populations. While resistance in zoonotic infections should be directly attributable to resistance in the zoonotic reservoir, the impact of agricultural antibiotic use remains controversial. Zoonotic species could acquire resistance genes from human commensal bacteria [a term given to all the natural bacteria that live on and in a healthy person] during the infection process, but this hypothesis is difficult to test.

For pathogens with high horizontal transmission rates, resistant bacteria will spread rapidly once they have emerged, and prevalence will be maintained at a steady state by horizontal transmission. Thus, the impact of subsequent heterospecific transmission is limited. Nevertheless, one or two heterospecific transmission events could be sufficient to cause the appearance of a highly successful ARB genotype in humans, affecting the timing, nature, and extent of spread within the human population. Not only are such events difficult to trace, but their impact is impossible to measure, since there is no way to know what type of resistance would have appeared and with what temporal pattern, if transfers from animals had been prevented.

The case where horizontal human transmission rates are intermediate is particularly interesting. If each case in a population generates approximately one new case (a situation we call "quasi-epidemic" transmission), each instance of heterospecific transmission will initiate a long chain of horizontal transmission that eventually burns out. Quasi-epidemic transmission can amplify a relatively low amount of heterospecific transmission and substantially increase prevalence. The effect is sustained as long as heterospecific transmission continues. A corollary is that banning agricultural antibiotic use would have maximal benefits if horizontal transmission is quasi-epidemic. Moreover, the effects are most difficult to estimate because both heterospecific and horizontal transmission must be accounted for.

These principles apply to bacteria associated with outpatient antibiotic use and community-acquired infections as well as those that are primarily hospital-acquired. Although quasi-epidemic transmission would seem to be a special case, it may in fact be the rule for many hospital-acquired bacteria because it is the natural endpoint of the interplay between economics and ecology. By spending money on hospital infection control, hospital administrators can reduce nosocomial [infections resulting from treatment in a hospital or other health care service unit but secondary to the patient's original condition] transmission rates for resistant bacteria. For example, hospitals may screen and isolate patients who are likely to be carriers (i.e., active surveillance) and implement infection-control measures, but this comes at the cost of isolating patients. Total costs are minimized by spending just enough to eliminate (or nearly eliminate) the pathogen; thus, quasi-epidemic transmission is the economic optimum.

The Community as a Reservoir for Resistance

Horizontal transmission is further complicated by population structure, such as the movement of humans through hospitals and long-term care facilities. Medical antibiotic use and horizontal transmission rates are high in hospitals, but this is counterbalanced by short hospital stays. An emerging view for hospital-acquired bacterial infections is that persistent asymptomatic carriage plays a key role in the epidemic of resistance. ARB can asymptomatically colonize a person for years: even if the number of other people infected during a single hospital visit is less than one, this number will exceed one when summed over several hospital visits. Thus, the ecological reservoir of resistance in the community plays an important role in the increasing frequency of resistance in hospital-acquired infections.

Short hospital visits and long persistence times of ARB in people guarantee that some of the costs associated with failed infection control are passed on to other hospitals—new carriers are frequently discharged from one hospital only to be admitted to another hospital later. Thus, the harm done by these ARB is borne by the whole human population, particularly all of the health-care institutions that serve a single catchment population. In economic terms, the damage caused by the carriage of ARB is a kind of pollution.

By comparing the total number of new carriers generated in the community, the impacts of agricultural antibiotic use on hospitals can be compared directly to the impact hospitals have on each other. The rate of heterospecific transmission is intrinsically difficult to measure directly because the risk of exposure and colonization per meal is very small. Nevertheless, agricultural antibiotic use may generate as many carriers as hospitals for the simple reason that the population experiences many more meals than hospital discharges. When agricultural and nosocomial transmission are equally rare in the population, the latter will be much easier to identify and quantify.

A Natural Experiment: Glycopeptides and Vancomycin-Resistant Enterococci

Is the impact of agricultural antibiotic use on the emergence and spread of ARB in humans large or small relative to medical antibiotic use? Put another way, are farms or hospitals bigger polluters? A large-scale natural experiment was conducted in the United States and several European countries when each adopted different policies on glycopeptide use in animals (avoparcin) and humans (vancomycin). Many European countries approved avoparcin for animal growth promotion in the 1970s, but the US did not.

In the early 1980s, demand for vancomycin in US hospitals surged because of increasing aminoglycoside resistance among enterococci and methicillin resistance in *Staphylococcus aureus*. Physicians in US hospitals also used oral vancomycin for some *Clostridium difficile* infections. In the late 1980s and early 1990s, vancomycin-resistant enterococci (VRE) emerged and spread through US health-care systems. In Europe, hospitals used less vancomycin because most enterococci were sensitive to aminoglycosides, and oral vancomycin was seldom used. VRE still emerged and spread through European hospitals, but the problem has been less severe than in the US.

A different pattern emerges for community prevalence of VRE. VRE are rarely found outside of hospitals in the US, except for patients who have a prior history of hospitalization. Community prevalence of VRE in the US is typically less than 1%. In contrast, community prevalence of VRE was estimated at 2%–12% in Europe during the late 1990s, including carriage by people with no history of hospitalization. In other words, the European community reservoir generated by vancomycin use in hospitals and avoparcin use in agriculture was apparently much larger than the US community reservoir generated only by vancomycin use in hospitals.

The prevalence of VRE in the community declined after the EU banned avoparcin. Thus, avoparcin is at least partly responsible for the reservoir of VRE in the European community, but how much of that reservoir came from avoparcin and how much came from hospitals? To weigh the impact, we subtract the community prevalence of VRE in the US from the community prevalence of VRE in Europe. The remainder is attributed to avoparcin. This analysis probably underestimates the real impact because vancomycin was used less in European than in US hospitals. Thus, avoparcin use in Europe would appear to be responsible for generating a larger reservoir of VRE in the community than US hospitals. Put another way, the impact of avoparcin use on European hospitals was larger than the impact of US hospitals on one another.

The EU banned the use of antibiotics for growth promotion, based on the precautionary principle.

Continuing Uncertainty and Need for Precaution

Despite the evidence that avoparcin use has had a large impact on the emergence and spread of VRE by increasing the reservoir of VRE in the EU, some uncertainty continues to surround the clinical significance of VRE strains of animal origin and of the zoonotic origins of resistance in general.

Bacterial strains circulating in hospitalized populations may be genetically distinct from those circulating in the general human population. Thus, bacterial populations are some combination of zoonotic, quasi-epidemic, and epidemic strains. The complexity of bacterial population biology and genetics makes it practically impossible to trace bacteria (or resistance factors) from the farm to the hospital, or to directly attribute some fraction of new infections to agricultural antibiotic use. Asymptomatic carriage of resistance factors by nonfocal commensal bacteria adds to a general risk of resistance, but transfer of resistance among bacterial species is unpredictable and difficult to quantify. Until more evidence is available, it is prudent and reasonable to consider bacteria with resistance genes a general threat.

The effects of agricultural antibiotic use on human health remain uncertain, despite extensive investigation, and the effects may be unknowable.

Some part of the controversy over agricultural antibiotic use has been a disagreement about how to weigh evidence and make decisions when the underlying biological processes are complex. In this case, the effects of agricultural antibiotic use on human health remain uncertain, despite extensive investigation, and the effects may be unknowable, unprovable, or immeasurable by the empirical standards of experimental biology. What should be done when complexity makes an important public-health effect intrinsically difficult to measure? What is an appropriate "null hypothesis" or its equivalent? Should the same standards of proof be used in science and science-based policy? Where should the burden of proof fall?

Scientific assessments for policy should summarize the best state of the science, recognizing that the burdens and standards of proof are necessarily softer because of the uncertainty that is introduced by biological complexity. The best decisions weigh the evidence in light of the inherent uncertainty. The EU banned the use of antibiotics for growth promotion, based on the precautionary principle. The use of the precautionary principle was criticized by some as unscientific in this context. In fact, the intrinsic problem of knowability, posed by the biological complexity of the problem, makes the use of precautionary decision making particularly suitable in this arena. The assumption that plausible dangers are negligible, even when it is known that such dangers are constitutively very difficult to measure, may be more unscientific than the use of precaution.

The Use of Antibiotics in Food Animals May Be the Main Source of Resistance in Food-Borne Pathogens

Union of Concerned Scientists

Union of Concerned Scientists *is a science-based nonprofit organization that works for a healthy environment and a safer world.*

If you get food poisoning, will the antibiotic prescribed by your doctor be able to fight the infection? This seems like an age of miracle drugs. Few weeks go by without a news story heralding a promising new drug or drug therapy. Ironically, concealed in the din of information about new drugs looms a health crisis growing out of the loss of old drugs.

Once a storehouse full of medicines such as penicillin and streptomycin could handily fight off most infections from bacteria and other microorganisms. Now, once-vulnerable bacteria have evolved resistance, and many of these drugs are losing their effectiveness. Health experts agree that there is serious danger of losing some of the most precious drugs—drugs that are most familiar as antibiotics, a subgroup of a larger group of threatened agents known as antimicrobials. Some strains of tuberculosis, for example, are now resistant to all available antimicrobial drugs. Unfortunately, tuberculosis is not the only resistant microorganism on the public health horizon.

Why are these drugs losing their power? Because they're being overused. Bacteria become resistant to antibiotics through overexposure to them. Hardy strains of the bacteria survive the exposure and pass on that resistance trait to successive generations. And they also pass the trait across to other bacteria that are unrelated, including some that cause human disease. Eventually the antibiotic wipes out all the vulnerable bacteria, and only resistant bacteria remain. Then the drug is no longer effective.

Preserving the effectiveness of antibiotics and other antimicrobials will require changes in all major areas of use: human medicine, veterinary medicine, and agriculture. But agricultural uses deserve special attention, since they provide resistant bacteria with a direct route into people's kitchens.

From Feedlot to Kitchen

Bacteria that become resistant in agricultural, particularly livestock, operations can be transferred to the general human population via food. According to a 1998 National Research Council study, *The Use of Drugs in Food Animals: Benefits and Risks*, the reported incidence of bacteria-related food-borne illness is increasing. The government is increasingly concerned about food-borne diseases caused by Campylobacter and Salmonella. As resistant strains of bacteria emerge, they have easy passage to humans—right though the grocery store.

> *The CDC has concluded that, in the United States, antimicrobial use in food animals is the dominant source of antibiotic resistance among food-borne pathogens.*

Campylobacter, for example, is carried into kitchens on poultry and can cause illness when people eat raw or undercooked poultry meat. While this does not always cause severe illness, the Centers for Disease Control and Prevention (CDC) estimate that there are two to four million Campylobacter infections per year, resulting in as many as 250 deaths each year in the United States. Furthermore, about one in a thousand Campylobacter infections leads to Guillan-Barre syndrome, a disease that can cause paralysis. Thus, the emergence of drug-resistant Campylobacter would be a serious public health concern.

In fact, Campylobacter is becoming resistant to the fluoroquinolones, a precious class of antibiotics, as a result of agricultural use. Only recently were fluoroquinolones approved for use in poultry in the United States. Before this use, no fluoroquinolone resistance was reported in people unless they had previously taken the drugs for illness or traveled to a country that permitted their use in agriculture. But now, resistant strains are emerging in samples taken from both humans and poultry. The correlation of the emergence of resistance with the use in animal systems is important evidence that agricultural use is the culprit.

Antimicrobial use in agriculture can also compromise human therapies when bacteria develop cross-resistance—when their resistance to one drug also makes them resistant to other, related drugs. This has happened in Europe with vancomycin, one of the drugs of last resort for treating certain life-threatening infections. Data suggest that rising levels of vancomycin-resistant bacteria in hospitals may have resulted from use in agriculture of avoparcin, a drug chemically related to vancomycin. Because avoparcin and vancomycin are similar in structure, bacteria resistant to avoparcin are resistant to vancomycin as well.

While some uses of antibiotics in livestock operations are a matter of animal health, other uses have an economic motive.

Similar phenomena are apparently occurring as a result of the use of antimicrobial drugs in the United States. The effectiveness of synercid, a drug of last resort for the treatment of vancomycin-resistant infections, is threatened because of the use of virginiamycin as a growth promoter in chickens and pigs in the United States. Virginiamycin is chemically related to synercid, so that bacteria resistant to the one drug also appear to be resistant to the other.

While the links between animal agriculture and human disease are complicated and in need of additional study, evidence is strong enough for scientists and public health organizations to call for reduced use of antimicrobial growth promoters in agriculture. The CDC has concluded that, in the United States, antimicrobial use in food animals is the dominant source of antibiotic resistance among food-borne pathogens.

Beefing Up Food

What can be done so that these drugs remain useful? Aren't antibiotics necessary to preserve the health of the livestock? While some uses of antibiotics in livestock operations are a matter of animal health, other uses have an economic motive. Especially troubling is their use not to cure sick animals but to promote "feed efficiency," that is, to increase the animal's weight gain per unit of feed. This so-called subtherapeutic use translates into relatively cheap meat prices at the grocery store.

But is this economic motive an essential use of these drugs? First, the economic advantage appears to be minimal. The National Research Council study estimated that a ban on such subtherapeutic use in livestock would increase per capita costs between $5 and $10 per year. That is a price most people would willingly pay to preserve a robust arsenal of medicines against infectious disease.

Second, using antimicrobial drugs is not the only way to lower meat costs. The same report suggests that adopting other methods of maintaining animal health, comfort, and well being could reduce drug use and cut costs. Such methods might include reducing overcrowding, controlling heat stress, providing vaccination to prevent disease, and using beneficial microbial cultures.

Reduction Problems

Although reducing or eliminating the use of antibiotics to promote growth is a straightforward solution to the problem of resistance, this will be difficult to achieve. Eliminating this use of antibiotics challenges the standard operating procedures of a large and powerful industry.

The subtherapeutic use of antibiotics is ingrained in livestock operations because it works. Chickens, cows, and pigs—particularly those that are not healthy to begin with—do gain weight faster when these drugs are added to their feed, and those gains translate into higher profits. In addition, livestock producers have bought into the myth that bacteria that cause illness in humans develop resistance only in medical settings. While no one denies that unwise use of antibiotics in human medicine is a source of serious resistance problems, this view has prevented recognition of one of the most attractive opportunities to cut back on these drugs—in subtherapeutic agricultural applications.

Obvious nonessential uses [of antibiotics], such as their ... use in livestock operations, should be the first target.

Agricultural use, much of it for growth promotion, accounts for 40 percent of the antibiotics sold in the United States. This enormous amount of drugs is delivered to animals under conditions congenial to the development of resistance. Large numbers of similar animals are raised in the concentrated facilities that characterize contemporary agriculture. Chicken houses, for example, can contain 20,000 birds. And the Environmental Protection Agency has identified 6,600 operations with at least 1,000 beef cattle or 700 dairy cattle or 2,500 hogs or 100,000 chickens.

In such large operations, antibiotics are often delivered to animals in food and water over extended periods. Bacteria are constantly being exposed to the drugs and eliminated from the populations. It is hard to imagine how resistance would not develop under these circumstances. Indeed, industrial livestock systems are hog heaven for resistant bacteria.

What's Next

The battle against emergence of antimicrobial resistance will take place on many fronts: in hospitals, in doctors' and veterinarians' offices, and on farms. The most sensible approach is to identify and reduce nonessential uses of antibiotics and reserve as many of these drugs as possible for wise use in human and veterinary medicine. Obvious nonessential uses, such as their subtherapeutic use in livestock operations, should be the first target in the effort to save antibiotics. Indeed, the CDC and the World Health Organization have called for an end to the use for growth promotion in animals of those drugs that are used to treat human disease or that are related to such medicines. UCS [Union of Concerned Scientists] is taking a careful look at the health risks of industrial agriculture and will be working to reduce the subtherapeutic use of antibiotics in livestock.

The U.S. Food and Drug Administration Ensures the Safe Use of Antibiotics in Animal Agriculture

Gary Weber

Gary Weber is executive director of Regulatory Affairs for the National Cattlemen's Beef Association, a trade group.

U.S. cattlemen care for their cattle by using government-approved antibiotics and other medications to prevent and treat diseases, similar to the way antibiotics are used to protect human health. More than 15 years ago, the cattle industry created its own quality assurance program that helps cattle producers and feedlot operators ensure these animal health products are used properly—and monitoring data show they are.

A History of Government Oversight

The Food and Drug Administration (FDA) first approved the sub-therapeutic and therapeutic use of antibiotics for farm animals in 1951. This use of antibiotics improved animal health by treating disease and improving animal productivity—ultimately resulting in greater production efficiency. The ability to treat animal diseases effectively helps cattle producers prevent animal suffering and ensure that only healthy cattle enter the human food chain.

Various antimicrobial compounds are used therapeutically, for relatively short periods of time, to treat and cure animals that are ill or at a high risk of becoming ill. Antibiotics may also be used sub-therapeutically, or at low levels, to aid animal

Gary Weber, "FDA Approvals Ensure Safe Antibiotic Use," *Issues Update-Beef Industry Publication*, May-June 2006. Reproduced with permission from The Cattlemen's Beef Board and The National Cattlemen's Beef Association.

growth and prevent bacterial disease from occurring. This is achieved by adding small amounts of antibiotics to feed or water. It helps control intestinal bacteria that could interfere with an animal's ability to absorb nutrients from feed and it helps control infections before they become a problem to the animal's health.

Most scientists agree that the improper use of antibiotics in human medicine is the greatest contributing factor in the formation of resistant bacteria affecting humans.

Managing Resistance Concerns

Some bacteria are inherently resistant to certain antibiotics, while others may develop resistance over time. However, most scientists agree that the improper use of antibiotics in human medicine is the greatest contributing factor in the formation of resistant bacteria affecting humans. Antibiotic use in animal agriculture makes a very small contribution to the resistance issue and in fact, all data indicate no resistance concerns are associated with beef products.

The availability and use of animal health products is obviously important to protect animal health, but equally important to protect animal well-being. Cattle producers also care about protecting public health and the future use of this important animal health management tool; so in the early 1990s, the Beef Quality Assurance program was created in response to concerns about developing antimicrobial resistance to antibiotics. This program educates cattle producers about the proper use of antibiotics, including making sure that withdrawal times are strictly observed when antibiotics are administered. Today, 98 percent of cattle going through feedlots and 90 percent of cattle on farms and ranches are from states with quality assurance programs in place. The principles followed by these operators are codified in the "Producer Guidelines for the Judicious Use of Antimicrobials in Cattle," which were developed in close cooperation with the American Association of Bovine Practitioners, the Academy of Veterinary Consultants and the American Veterinary Medical Association.

The government also addresses antibiotic resistance concerns through FDA's "Guidance for Industry Part 152." Guidance 152 is a tool for animal health companies to use as they develop potential antimicrobials. This guidance outlines the recommended methods for ensuring any proposed antimicrobial product is analyzed for risk of resistance development that could potentially affect public health. In addition, any antimicrobial proposed for FDA approval is reviewed by an independent group of experts on the FDA's Veterinary Medical Advisory Committee (VMAC). Many sources of data, including the U.S. Department of Agriculture (USDA) Food Safety Inspection Service (FSIS) residue monitoring program, continue to show that there is no evidence of antibiotic residue violations associated with beef production.

Risk assessments determine product future. FDA has approved two products in the class of antibiotics known as flouroquinilones. The approval was based on risk analysis, which shows the use of these products to treat cattle diseases like pneumonia, will present little, if any, public health risk. One element of that risk analysis evaluated whether using these products could increase the risk of antibiotic resistance to flouroquinilones in selected foodborne pathogens, because flouroquinilones may be used to treat such infections in people under certain conditions. The risk analysis showed that, based upon the patterns of use and other factors, these antibiotics do not represent a public health risk when used to treat cattle for disease conditions.

A Link Between Agricultural Use of Antibiotics and Resistant Infections Has Not Been Proven

Dale W. Rozeboom, Barbara E. Straw, Hui Li, and David K. Beede

Dale W. Rozeboom is state swine specialist at the Department of Animal Science at Michigan State University (MSU). Also from MSU, Barbara E. Straw is extension swine veterinarian, Large Animal Clinical Science; Hui Li is assistant professor, Crop and Soil Science; and David K. Beede is Meadows Chair, Department of Animal Science. The article was originally published as a factsheet for the Gratiot County (Mich.) Livestock Forums.

We share the world with a wide range of living organisms from microscopic bacteria to gigantic whales. Although we cannot see them, bacteria are all around us and are a normal part of our ecosystem and lives. Different kinds of bacteria are in competition with each other for nutrients and living space. Bacteria are specialized and fill various niches in the environment. For example, the soil is full of bacteria that live off of soil nutrients, moisture and decaying material. Other bacteria live best in the bodies of people and animals, benefiting them, while others cause disease.

Antibiotics and Resistance

Some soil bacteria naturally produce substances (antibiotics or antimicrobials) that inhibit the growth of other bacteria. Scientists cultivate these soil bacteria and collect the antibiotics produced. The antibiotic may be given to people to help fight infections or disease caused by other bacteria. Not all bacteria are affected the same way by the specific type of antibiotic. While the growth of non-resistant bacteria is suppressed, resistant bacteria can continue to live in the presence of antibiotics. Resistance is the inherent ability of some bacteria to resist being killed by an antibiotic. Resistance was present prior to the use of antibiotics and occurs as a result of genetic mutation or when extra chromosomal DNA (plasmid) is acquired from other bacteria. In theory, antibiotic use selects for resistant bacteria, allowing them to multiply without the competition of antibiotic-susceptible bacteria.

Antimicrobials are used in human medicine and animal agriculture to reduce disease and death.

The literal meaning of the word antibiotic, used commonly for decades, is "against life." It is less precise than the term "antimicrobial" which means "against microbes." ... [Here] the two names are used interchangeably despite the scientifically more accurate meaning of the term antimicrobial.

Antimicrobials are used in human medicine and animal agriculture to reduce disease and death. They are given by injection, orally, and in food and water to prevent or treat diseases, and as growth promoters. Exact amounts currently manufactured and used are not available.

Antibiotics used for growth promotion [in livestock], lessen the effects of sub-clinical disease, thus food consumption, weight gain, and the efficiency of food use for growth are improved. They are not effective when disease is absent.

Antibiotics in the Environment

What about antibiotics from livestock production entering the environment? Will antibiotics used in livestock production have a negative impact on ground or surface water?

Chemicals used in homes, manufacturing, and agriculture can enter the environment in wastewater. A 1999 study by the Toxic Substances Hydrology Program of the U.S. Geological Survey [USGS] found a range of chemicals in residential, industrial and agricultural wastewaters and at low concentrations in surface waters. The chemicals included human and veterinary pharmaceuticals (including antibiotics), natural and synthetic hormones, detergent metabolites, plasticizers, insecticides, and fire retardants. Measured concentrations of pharmaceuticals in wastewaters were much lower than would be found if a person or animal were consuming the chemical. Most are detected in water at concentrations less than 1 microgram per liter. These amounts are relatively small compared to the dosage provided to humans and animals to treat disease. For example, the antibiotic tetracycline may be given to humans at a rate of 2 grams per day, usually in 2 to 4 pills taken orally. If given to pigs as a growth promoter, the dosage is 0.05 grams per day. Higher concentrations occurred in sediments because of sorption. In Huron County, Michigan, a USGS study found both human-use and veterinary-use antibiotics in stream (surface) water, but not in groundwater. Whether these findings are of biological, environmental or health consequence are currently unknown. Research is being proposed and conducted.

Up to 40% or more of the antibiotic dose may be excreted, especially for antibiotics given at therapeutic doses. This is true for both humans and animals. However, different classes of antibiotics are more or less metabolized. Antibiotics are excreted in urine and feces either unchanged or metabolized in the form of the conjugated, oxidized or hydrolyzed products of parent compounds.

Antibiotics may enter the environment in wastewater, or when human waste solids and animal manures are applied to cropland as plant fertilizer. Some antibiotics degrade quite slowly, possibly surviving the processes of storage and handling, and may be present in land-applied biosolids. The continual land application of bio-solids could cause the rates of antibiotic accumulation in soils to exceed the rates of degradation. However, accumulation in soils is less probable as environmental regulations and voluntary generally accepted management practices limit manure application so that applied nutrients meet the requirement of the crop being grown.

The incidence of human disease caused by antibiotic-resistant organisms is not greater in people working on livestock farms as compared with those who do not.

Understanding the fate and transport of antibiotics in the environment is essential to assess their impact and subsequent risks to ecosystems. Sorption (absorption or to take up; and adsorption or to hold) by soil plays a determinant role in controlling transport, bioavailability and hence fate of antibiotics in the environment. The complicated chemical structures of antibiotics lead to multiple interactions with soils. In general, soil organic matter and minerals are the two soil components responsible for holding antibiotics. A few studies have attempted to address the sorption mechanisms, but so far they are far from being fully understood. . . .

The Link Between Agriculture and Resistant Human Infections

[A] link between agricultural use of antimicrobials and antibiotic-resistant human infections has not been proven, only speculated. The incidence of human disease caused by antibiotic resistant organisms is not greater in people working on livestock farms as compared with those who do not. In the past, cases of what was believed initially to be resistant bacteria from animals spreading to man were headlined in the press. But when these potential examples were examined closely, other more usual risk factors (such as antibiotics already in people before infection or a hospital stay) were present and much more of a health risk.

Antibiotic resistance can occur in bacteria even when the antibiotics have not been used.

Antibiotics have been used in animals over 60 years. However, antibiotic resistance only recently has become a major medical concern in hospitals. Whenever a population of bacteria, of importance to animals or humans, is exposed to an antibiotic it encourages the predominance of the most resistant strains of the bacteria. The most well-known example of this is how rapidly gonorrhea became resistant to penicillin. It is possible for resistant bacteria from animals to make their way into humans, but many barriers stand in their way. Most bacteria that cause animal diseases are specialized for that species (species-specific) and poorly invade humans. Zoonotic bacteria, such as certain species of Escherichia coli and Salmonella are of greater concern as they are transmissible from animals to humans. Usual precautions of washing hands and thoroughly cooking of foods eliminate the spread of these to humans, but these procedures do not help prevent environmental transmission (e.g., to drinking water).

Antibiotic resistance can occur in bacteria even when the antibiotics have not been used. Researchers found tetracycline- and tylosin-resistant bacteria in manure samples taken from storage facilities of swine farms where antimicrobials were not being used. Likewise, ... resistance of E. coli to tetracycline, sulfonamides and streptomycin was similarly prevalent in feces of broiler chickens both receiving and not receiving antibiotics. [Researchers] ... also reported that tetracycline and tylosin resistant bacteria were isolated in soil of fields where manure was applied "regularly" and in the feces of dogs kept as pets on the farm. But, the prevalence of resistant bacteria did not differ among farms using or not using antimicrobials as a feed additive for growth promotion.

Bacteria have complex genetic means for transferring resistance. Some scientists hypothesize that cause (antibiotic use) and effect (antibiotic resistance) may be linked. Doubtless, detailed exploration of microbial genetics will evaluate this suggestion in the future.

Banning use of antimicrobials for growth promotion [in agriculture] did not affect the incidence of . . . [resistant] infections in humans.

Banning or Reducing Agricultural Use of Antibiotics

[Discontinuing the use of antibiotics for growth promotion and disease prevention to decrease the risks associated with using antibiotics in animal agriculture] was the thinking in Denmark and some European countries where use of low levels of many antibiotics in livestock was banned. Monitoring the prevalence of antibiotic resistant bacteria in animal manure found lower numbers after the ban. The designers of the antibiotic ban used this finding to claim success. However, when examining a more immediate outcome such as the level of resistant infections in people the results were not clear. The animals raised for food in these countries now have a lower health status and their mortality rate has increased. Because of the lower health status, it is more expensive to raise food and the incidence of resistant infections affecting people has not decreased. Total antimicrobial use has decreased slightly, but therapeutic usage has surpassed growth promoter usage prior to the ban. Banning use of antimicrobials for growth promotion did not affect the incidence of antimicrobial residues in foods or the incidence of Salmonella, Campylobacter, or Yersinia infections in humans.

It is [also] very difficult to conclude that animal health is related to size of the farm. There have been no controlled studies evaluating this. Retrospective data suggest that this is true, if one assumes that the amount of antibiotic use is correlated positively with the amount of disease. A [2002] survey conducted by the National Animal Health Monitoring System [NAHMS] found that 78% of farms with 2,000 or less pigs used feed-grade antibiotics as compared with 94% of farms with 10,000 or more. However in 2005, NAHMS released a report on dairy farming documenting that a greater percentage of large (500 or more cows) and medium-sized (100 to 499 cows) operations fed antimicrobials in heifer (pre-lactation) rations than did small (less than 100 cows) operations (36%, 30% and 15%, respectively). Note that antibiotics that might appear in milk are not approved for feeding to lactating dairy cows. Antibiotics are not allowed to be present in milk for public sale according to the Federal [U.S. Food and] Drug Administration's Grade A Pasteurized Milk Ordinance under the Federal Food, Drug and Cosmetic Act. Similar percentages of small (1,000 to 7,999 head) and large (8,000 head or more) beef feedlots practice antimicrobial feeding and (or) watering. However, the assumption that the amount of antibiotic use and the amount of disease may be related may not be valid because large farms have better record keeping systems and make greater use of veterinary services and disease diagnostics. Simply, there are more accurate data and greater veterinary use on large farms for reasons other than disease occurrence alone.

There Must Be More Study of the Risk to Public Health from Agricultural Use of Antibiotics

Scott A. McEwen

Scott A. McEwen is a doctor of veterinary medicine and a professor in the Department of Population Medicine at the Ontario Veterinary College in Guelph, Ontario.

"Superbugs", bacteria resistant to all or nearly all of the antibiotics available to doctors, have received a lot of press lately. It's scary to think that common infections that we are used to treating with antibiotics may someday be untreatable, but in some cases that may soon happen. Some important bacteria, such as methicillin-resistant Staphylococcus aureus and vancomycin-resistant enterococci are already resistant to all but a very few antibiotics. And development of new classes of antibiotics by the pharmaceutical industry has slowed to a trickle.

Health Effects of Non-Human Uses of Antibiotics

It's been shown in many countries that antibiotic-prescribing practices in hospitals and the community can often be directly linked to emergence of resistance. But what about non-human uses of antibiotics? We use antibiotics to treat bacterial infections in animals, including fish, farm animals and pets. But antibiotics are also extensively used to prevent disease and to promote growth in food animals. In some countries, antibiotics are also used for prevention of bacterial infections of fruit.

How does the human health impact of these non-human uses stack up? The evidence suggests that antibiotic use and

Scott A. McEwen, "Drugs and Bugs: The Widespread Use of Antibiotics in Agriculture May Build Resistant Bacteria and Affect Our Ability to Treat Human Disease," *Alternatives Journal*, vol. 31.3, 2005, pp. 22–23. Copyright © 2005 Alternatives, Inc. Reproduced by permission of the publisher and author. Subscriptions at www.alternativesjournal.ca.

abuse in humans drives resistance among the foremost respiratory, genital, urinary and skin infections. On the other hand, antibiotic use in agriculture is thought to have an impact largely on the human intestinal infections for which animals are important sources (for example zoonoses—diseases that are passed from animals to humans—such as Salmonella and Campylobacter). Since plants and farmed fish are infrequent sources of intestinal bacteria for humans, most of the attention has focused on antibiotic use in terrestrial animals.

In Canada and many other countries, thousands of intestinal infections are passed from animals to humans through contaminated food and water. These agents are pathogenic to humans whether or not they are resistant to antibiotics. Therefore to assess the impact of resistance on human health it is necessary to estimate any extra burden of illness attributable to resistance.

In food-borne infections, antibiotic resistance can have multiple effects on human health. Resistance can render infections more difficult or expensive to treat, or produce more severe or longer-lasting disease through enhanced virulence or pathogenicity. And because antibiotics also kill healthy flora in the gut that protect against illness, resistance can also increase the risk of infection (of Salmonella in particular) in people taking antibiotics for other reasons.

Because of the complexity of the farm-to-fork continuum, it is difficult to study the public health risks associated with non-human uses of antibiotics directly.

Furthermore, evolutionary processes of selection and adaptation can increase the pool of resistant genes in our ecosystem, and promote their spread among different species of bacteria. And when animals undergo antibiotic therapy, increased resistance to antibiotics can enhance the spread of zoonotic infections among the animals themselves, making them more likely to spread to humans by direct or indirect means.

The Magnitude of the Risk

While there is qualitative evidence that antibiotic use in agriculture contributes to resistance in human infections, only a few estimates of the magnitude of this contribution have been published. Many national bodies that regulate veterinary drugs, as well as the World Health Organization and other international agencies, are currently grappling with how best to assess the risks in order to be able to make reasonable regulatory decisions that address those risks. It is also important to consider the benefits of antibiotics to animal health, animal welfare and animal production.

Because of the complexity of the farm-to-fork continuum, it is difficult to study the public health risks associated with non-human uses of antibiotics directly. Therefore, indirect means of studying these risks must be found. Fortunately, through targeted research studies and surveillance programs, we know a lot more about the issue than we did just a few years ago.

We need to learn much more about antibiotic resistance in the food chain ... and the increased virulence of these bacteria in humans.

In some countries (notably Denmark) special surveillance systems have provided crucial information on the relationships between various types of antibiotic use in animals and resistance in animals, food and humans. They have allowed us to learn more about the effects that changes in antibiotic-use policies (e.g., the banning of antibiotic growth promoters) have had on resistance, food safety, animal production, and animal and human health.

Other countries are following suit. Improved surveillance of resistance and antibiotic use in Canada were among the recommendations made by recent national expert panels and the Canadian Integrated Program for Antibiotic Resistance Surveillance released its first report (on 2002 data) in March 2004.

There is also reason for optimism that food safety programs and on-farm quality assurance programs will reduce the spread of bacteria from food animals to humans through contaminated food products. Similar general efforts to control the contamination of drinking water by farm-origin bacteria also provide reasons for optimism. There are, of course, challenges ahead. Food and water safety programs as well as on-farm quality assurance programs must be designed to explicitly consider antibiotic resistance. Veterinarians and farmers also must be convinced to take the issue seriously.

We need to learn much more about antibiotic resistance in the food chain—its emergence, spread, persistence and factors that might affect its decline. We also need to study intently the association between antibiotic resistance and the increased virulence of these bacteria in humans. Uncertainties abound in this field and research is critical to preserving these valuable drugs.

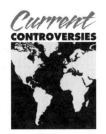

CHAPTER 3

Are Drug Companies at Fault for Not Developing Better Antibacterial Drugs?

Chapter Preface

Many experts believe the key to winning the war against resistant infections is researching and developing new types of antibiotics or other drugs to wipe out the new, drug-resistant types of bacteria. However, because most of the major pharmaceutical companies have pulled out of antibiotic research in favor of more profitable types of drug research, small drug companies appear to be the best hope for new antibiotic drugs.

In fact, although thirteen new antibiotic drugs have reached the market since 1998, only one—CUBICIN, produced by a small company, Cubist Pharmaceuticals—has been truly effective and successful. CUBICIN was developed and marketed starting in 2003 as a treatment for serious skin infections that can develop after surgery. In 2006, the drug also was approved for the treatment of bloodstream infections caused by catheters, surgery, or intravenous drug usage. The drug is effective against methicillin-resistant *Staphylococcus aureus* (MRSA), as well as a broad range of other bacteria, including *Streptococcus pyogenes*, *S. agalactiae*, *S. dysgalactiae subsp equisimilis*, and vancomycin-resistant *Enterococcus faecalis*. According to the company Web site, the active pharmaceutical ingredient in CUBICIN—daptomycin—is a natural product that is produced by *Streptomyces roseosporus*, a microorganism found in the soil. It works in a novel way—by binding to and penetrating the cell membrane of bacteria, causing cell death. CUBICIN so far has reaped more than $320 million in sales for Cubist, and annual revenue is expected to reach $200 million by the end of 2008.

However, small companies such as Cubist face formidable development obstacles in bringing new antibiotic products to the market. It is estimated that it takes five to eight years of research to discover and develop a new drug product, and still another five to eight years to win approval from the U.S. Food and Drug Administration (FDA) to market the drug. Drug companies, therefore, have to be able to predict future drug needs at least a decade ahead of when the need might arise. And the costs of such development and marketing efforts can be huge. According to Cubist's managers, for example, the company will not begin to make a profit on CUBICIN until it recovers $490 million it spent on research and development. Cubist hopes to win approval to market the drug for still other uses, including lung infections and hospital-acquired diarrhea, and over the long run, CUBICIN is expected to be profitable for the company. Despite the prospect of such success, however, companies could experience major losses if they expend large sums to develop antibiotics that fail to produce enough sales to cover expenses.

In the future, some experts predict that demand for treatments of drug-resistant bacteria will rise as the number of infections grow, the number of deaths increases, and health care costs continue to rise. A few biotech companies, including Basilea, Oceint, and Paratek, are reportedly already working on new classes of antibiotics to meet this expected demand, but none has yet received FDA approval. If demand increases further, more companies may decide to enter the field.

Federal government incentives also may help to encourage more antibiotic drug development. Already, hundreds of millions of dollars have been made available in the form of research grants to support research on drugs to protect against bioterrorism agents such as plague and anthrax, and some experts have suggested that such research also may result in products that control drug-resistant infectious diseases. In addition, the U.S. government has been under increasing pressure to create financial and regulatory incentives for major drug companies to return to development of antibiotic drugs. For example, the FDA has a mechanism by which new drugs for the treatment of antibiotic-resistant infections can qualify for Orphan Drug status—a classification that entitles the drug company to government funding of clinical trials, one of the main expenses of new drug development. Finally, certain philanthropic organizations, such as the Global TB Alliance and the Bill and Melinda Gates Foundation, have donated funds to help develop new drugs to treat several drug-resistant diseases, including tuberculosis and malaria, affecting the developing world.

Despite these promising signs, most health experts say there remains an inadequate amount of investment in antibiotic research today. The viewpoints in this chapter address the critical issue of the drug companies' role in developing better antibacterial drugs.

The Major Drug Companies Are No Longer Researching Antibacterial Drugs

Guy Charron

Guy Charron is a Canadian writer for the World Socialist Web Site, *which opposes capitalism and promotes world socialism.*

Infectious disease specialists have drawn a causal link between an alarming rise in the number of Quebec hospital patients becoming infected with and dying from *Clostridium difficile*—a bacterium resistant to standard antibiotics—and government budget-cutting. As the *World Socialist Web Site* previously reported, researchers studying the *C. difficile* pandemic in Quebec have linked the bacteria's spread to the unsanitary environment created by decaying infrastructure, patient overcrowding, and reduced staffing.

The Threat of Superbugs

Hospital-based infections and bacteria resistant to standard antibiotics—so-called superbugs—are interlinked and growing problems. In Quebec, more than 3,000 people died last year [2003] as the result of infections they contracted while hospitalized, making hospital-contracted infections the fourth most important cause of death in Quebec. While many of the victims were persons who were very old or already seriously ill, a significant number succumbed to bacteria resistant to common antibiotics.

Since the early 1980s, the problem of superbugs has increasingly preoccupied medical specialists and with good reason. It is estimated that currently 20 percent of all bacterial infections in the US involve microbes resistant to one or more antibiotics.

Guy Charron, "As Superbug Problem Mounts, Drug Companies Slash Antibiotics Research," *World Socialist Web Site*, September 11, 2004. Reproduced by permission.

Media reports on the superbug phenomenon typically treat it as exclusively a natural phenomenon. Bacteria that are resistant to antibiotics or that have become resistant due to a mutation survive antibiotic treatments, while the elimination of the non-resistant strain facilitates the rapid proliferation of the "superbug." This explanation, based on the Darwinian principle of natural selection, is certainly scientifically valid. But like the spread of Quebec's *C. difficile*, the related general problem of superbugs is also linked to social conditions—poverty, the lack of basic hygiene, and the subordination of fundamental health care concerns to the profit needs of big business.

Despite the threat posed by bacteria resistant to standard antibiotics, the major pharmaceutical companies are withdrawing from research into antimicrobial drugs.

An article published almost 10 years ago [mid-1990s] in one of the journals of the American College of Physicians observed that in Asia, the Middle East and Latin America, home to more than three quarters of the world's population, there is the greatest concentration of antibiotic resistant bacteria, even though only 20 percent of all antibiotics are consumed there.

The article asked, "Why do countries that can afford so little have so great a problem with resistance to antimicrobial drugs? The situation appears to be due to a combination of a heavy burden of bacterial infectious diseases; huge populations without even the rudiments of primary health care; inappropriate use of the available antimicrobial drugs; and rapid spread through crowding, poor sanitation, and sexual contact. Self-prescribing is common in most developing countries, and the effect is compounded by a bewildering array of proprietary drugs containing irrational mixtures of vitamins, stimulants, and steroids and by the availability of drugs without prescription for purchase in local pharmacies or open-air markets. Physicians, when available, need to see as many patients as possible in the shortest period of time with minimal, if any, laboratory or radiologic support. They often feel compelled to prescribe antimicrobial drugs to meet patient expectations. The pharmacies work on small mark-ups. The amount of an antimicrobial purchased is often inadequate to treat serious infections. . . . In some countries, the political systems are so corrupt, the local business community so venal, and the physicians so disillusioned that the situation seems hopeless."

In 2001, Eli Lilly and Bristol-Myers Squibb stopped work on developing new antimicrobial drugs. Other major drug companies are reported to be about to do likewise.

A Lack of New Antibiotic Drugs

Nevertheless, the author still held out hope that the spread of superbugs could be reversed by the development of new antibiotics and other antimicrobial drugs. However, the situation has changed dramatically over the past decade. Despite the threat posed by bacteria resistant to standard antibiotics, the major pharmaceutical companies are withdrawing from research into antimicrobial drugs.

The number of new antimicrobial drugs approved by the FDA [Food and Drug Administration], the US agency responsible for authorizing the marketing of pharmaceuticals, has fallen significantly: 16 were approved between 1983 and 1987; 14 between 1988 and 1992; 10 between 1993 and 1997; and 10 more in the last five-year period, 1998–2003. In 2003, the number of new anti-infection agents submitted to the FDA [U.S. Food and Drug Administration] for testing fell by 10 percent from the year before, an indication that the long-term trend is likely to continue.

In 2001, Eli Lilly and Bristol-Myers Squibb stopped work on developing new antimicrobial drugs. Other major drug companies are reported to be about to do likewise. A major conference of microbiologists, doctors and pharmacists held in Chicago in September 2003 hosted a session devoted to discussing why the major drug companies are withdrawing from antibiotics and antimicrobial research. The session was titled "Why Is Big Pharma Getting Out of Anti-infective Drug Discovery?"

Because they can make larger profits by developing other sorts of drugs, the pharmaceutical companies are cutting back on antibacteria research.

Dr. Henry Masur, one of the session speakers, left no doubt as to the impact of drug makers' bottom-line on research decisions that will ultimately affect the lives of masses of people: "The cost of drug development is astronomical, the market is not nearly as enticing as markets that involve drugs that must be taken for a lifetime rather than days or weeks, and there is considerable pressure to reduce prices."

Nature, one of the world's leading scientific journals, summarized the Chicago session. Its summary read, in part: "Big drug companies are in the financial doldrums, and antibiotics research is easy to cut, said Steven Projan, who directs such work at Wyeth's facility in Pearl River, New York. Natural selection makes resistance inevitable, rendering any antibiotic less profitable over time. New drugs that combat resistant bacteria are often held in reserve by doctors to treat only the most stubborn infections—so they aren't big earners. And unlike drugs for chronic illnesses such as heart disease, antibiotics cure people, eliminating their customers."

Antibiotic sales are valued at between $24 and $26 billion per year and are expected to rise by 10 percent over the next four years. Yet, because they can make larger profits by developing other sorts of drugs, the pharmaceutical companies are cutting back on antibacteria research.

To evaluate the quality of an investment, the pharmaceutical industry uses an index called risk-adjusted net present value or NPV. It takes into account several factors, including expected sales, research costs and costs of the clinical tests needed to get government approval for mass marketing. According to the aforementioned [Dr.] Projan, antibiotics have an NPV of 100, anti-cancer drugs 300, neurological drugs 720 and muscular-skeletal 1150.

The pharmaceutical companies have replied to the criticism of their research decisions by complaining about the costs associated with getting government approval to market new antibiotics. Their standard refrain is that there is too much bureaucracy. FDA records show, however, that since 1964 anti-infection agents have had the highest approval rate of all classes of therapeutics and since 1982 the shortest or second shortest development time.

Drug Industry Economics Are at the Root of the Resistant Infection Problem

Sabin Russell

Sabin Russell is a medical writer for The San Francisco Chronicle, *a daily U.S. newspaper.*

At a busy microbiology lab in San Francisco, bad bugs are brewing inside vials of human blood, or sprouting inside petri dishes, all in preparation for a battery of tests.

These tests will tell doctors at UCSF [University of California San Francisco] Medical Center which kinds of bacteria are infecting their patients, and which antibiotics have the best chance to knock those infections down.

With disturbing regularity, the list of available options is short, and it is getting shorter.

The Problem of Drug-Resistant Infections

Dr. Jeff Brooks has been director of the UCSF lab for 29 years, and has watched with a mixture of fascination and dread how bacteria once tamed by antibiotics evolve rapidly into forms that practically no drug can treat.

"These organisms are very small," he said, "but they are still smarter than we are."

Among the most alarming of these is MRSA, or methicillin-resistant Staphylococcus aureus, a bug that used to be confined to vulnerable hospital patients, but now is infecting otherwise healthy people in schools, gymnasiums and the home.

As MRSA continues its natural evolution, even more drug-resistant strains are emerging. The most aggressive of these is one called USA300. . . .

[In January 2008], doctors at San Francisco General Hospital reported that a variant of that strain, resistant to six important antibiotics normally used to treat staph, may be transmitted by sexual contact and is spreading among gay men in San Francisco, Boston, New York and Los Angeles.

Yet the problem goes far beyond one bug and a handful of drugs. Entire classes of mainstay antibiotics are being threatened with obsolescence, and bugs far more dangerous than staph are evolving in ominous ways.

The supply of new antibiotics from drug company laboratories is running dry.

"We are on the verge of losing control of the situation, particularly in the hospitals," said Dr. Chip Chambers, chief of infectious disease at San Francisco General Hospital.

The reasons for increasing drug resistance are well known:

- Overuse of antibiotics, which speeds the natural evolution of bacteria, promoting new mutant strains resistant to those drugs.

- Careless prescribing of antibiotics that aren't effective for the malady in question, such as a viral infection.

- Patient demand for antibiotics when they aren't needed.

- Heavy use of antibiotics in poultry and livestock feed, which can breed resistance to similar drugs for people.

- Germ strains that interbreed at hospitals, where infection controls as simple as hand-washing are lax.

The Lack of New Antibiotics

All this is happening while the supply of new antibiotics from drug company laboratories is running dry.

Since commercial production of penicillin began in the 1940s, antibiotics have been the miracle drugs of modern medicine, suppressing infectious diseases that have afflicted human beings for thousands of years. But today, as a generation of Baby Boomers begins to enter a phase of life marked by the ailments of aging, we are running out of miracles.

Top infectious disease doctors are saying that lawmakers and the public at large do not realize the grave implications of this trend.

The strategy for nearly 70 years has been to stay a step ahead of resistance by developing new antibiotics ... [but] major drugmakers have been dropping out of the field.

"Within just a few years, we could be seeing that most of our microorganisms are resistant to most of our antibiotics," said Dr. Jack Edwards, chief of infectious diseases at Harbor-UCLA [University of California Los Angeles] Medical Center.

At Brooks' microbiology laboratory, the evolutionary struggle of bacteria versus antibiotics is on display every day. He grabbed a clear plastic dish that grew golden-hued MRSA germs taken from a patient a few days earlier. Inside were seven paper dots, each impregnated with a different drug. If the antibiotic worked, the dot had a clear ring around it—a zone where no germs could grow. No ring meant the drug had failed. This test was typical. Three drugs worked, four had failed.

The strategy for nearly 70 years has been to stay a step ahead of resistance by developing new antibiotics. In the past decade, however, major drugmakers have been dropping out of the field. The number of new antibiotics in development has plummeted. During the five-year period ended in 1987, the FDA [U.S. Food and Drug Administration] licensed 16 novel antibiotics. In the most recent five-year period, only five were approved.

For drugmakers, the economics are simple: An antibiotic can cure an infection in a matter of days. There is much more money in finding drugs that must be taken for a lifetime.

Each year 99,000 Americans die of various bacterial infections that they pick up while hospitalized—more than double the number killed . . . in automobile accidents.

Toll of Antibiotic Resistance

With antibiotic research lagging, the bugs are catching up, and infections are taking a terrible toll. The federal Centers for Disease Control and Prevention [CDC] estimates that each year 99,000 Americans die of various bacterial infections that they pick up while hospitalized—more than double the number killed every year in automobile accidents.

Of the 1.7 million hospital-acquired infections that occur each year, studies show, 70 percent are resistant to at least one antibiotic.

Drug-resistant staph is rapidly becoming a major public health menace. Last fall, the CDC estimated that MRSA alone has killed 19,000 Americans. Most of these patients picked up the bug in the hospital, but it is now spreading in urban and suburban neighborhoods across the nation.

"MRSA is killing people. It almost killed me," said Peg McQueary, whose life was upended when she nicked her leg with a razor three years ago.

Within days, her leg was grotesquely swollen, red from foot to knee. Her husband wheeled her into a Kaiser medical office, where her doctor took one look and rushed her to an isolation room.

She was placed on intravenous vancomycin, a drug reserved for the most serious cases of MRSA. Since that frightening week, the 42-year-old Roseville [Calif.] woman has spent much of her life in and out of hospitals, and she's learned just how difficult these infections can be to treat. Mc-Queary has burned through drug after drug, but the staph keeps coming back.

She's been hooked up at her home to bags of vancomycin and swallowed doses of linezolid, clindamycin and a half a dozen other antibiotics with barely pronounceable names and limited effect.

Drug-resistant staph is rapidly becoming a major public health menace.

One of the newest antibiotics, intravenous daptomycin—approved by the Food and Drug Administration [FDA] in 2003—seems to work the best, but it has not prevented recurrences.

"It's just a struggle to do everyday things," she said. "I am ready to scream about it."

Today, she moderates a Web site, MRSA Resources Support Forum, swapping stories with other sufferers. "Giving them a place to vent is some sort of healing for me," she said.

McQueary's travails are becoming an all-too-familiar American experience. As bacteria evolve new ways to sidestep antibiotics, doctors treating infections find themselves with a dwindling list of options. Old-line drugs are losing their punch, while the newer ones are both costly and laden with side effects.

The Weakening Grip of the Drugs

Dr. Joseph Guglielmo, chairman of the Department of Clinical Pharmacy at UCSF, closely tracks the effectiveness of dozens of antibiotics against different infectious bacteria. Laminated color-coded cards called antibiograms are printed up for hospital physicians each year. They chart the success rate of each antibiotic against at least 12 major pathogens. These charts show how antibiotics, like tires slowly leaking air, are losing strength year by year.

As head of the hospital pharmacy, Guglielmo oversees a small warehouse at the medical center that stores millions of dollars worth of prescription drugs that are used every day to treat patients there. Strolling down the aisles that house bins of antibiotics, he reached for a bottle of imipenem, and cradled the little vial in the palm of his hand.

"This one is the last line of defense," he said.

Imipenem was approved by the FDA in 1985. A powerful member of the carbapenem family—the latest in a long line of penicillin-like drugs—it is frequently used in hospitals today because it can still defeat a wide variety of germs that have outwitted the earlier-generation antibiotics.

But at a cost of about $60 a day, and with a safety profile that includes risk of seizure, it is a "Big Gun" drug that must be used carefully. As soon as doctors discover that a lesser antibiotic will work, they will stop prescribing imipenem, like soldiers conserving their last remaining stores of ammunition.

Now, there are signs of trouble.

Imipenem has been the antibiotic of choice for doctors treating Klebsiella, a vigorous microbe that causes pneumonia in hospitalized patients. But in June 2005, New York City doctors reported in the journal *Archives of Internal Medicine* outbreaks of imipenem-resistant Klebsiella. Fifty-nine such cases were logged at just two hospitals. The death rate among those whose infections entered their bloodstreams was 47 percent.

Last year [2007], Israeli doctors battled an outbreak of carbapenem-resistant Klebsiella that has killed more than 400 patients.

Cipro's Dramatic Decline

The antibiotic Cipro, approved by the Food and Drug Administration in 1987, is familiar to millions of Americans because it is widely prescribed for pneumonia, urinary tract infections and sexually transmitted diseases. It was the drug used to treat victims of the anthrax mailings that followed the Sept. 11, [2001] attacks.

Unlike most antibiotics, which originated from natural toxins produced by bacteria, Cipro came from tinkering with a chemical compound used to fight malaria. The German drug giant Bayer patented Cipro's active ingredient in 1983, and it subsequently became the most widely sold antibiotic in the world.

At hospitals across the country, however, clinicians have witnessed a remarkable drop-off in the utility of Cipro against more commonly encountered germs.

Antibiograms from the UCSF lab highlight the alarming erosion: As recently as 1999, Cipro was effective against 95 percent of specimens of E. coli—bacteria responsible for the most common hospital-acquired infections in the United States. By 2006, Cipro would work against only 60 percent of samples tested.

Other Antibiotics with Declining Effectiveness

The bacterial evolution that has so quickly sapped Cipro has also reduced the effectiveness of the entire family of related antibiotics called fluoroquinolones—drugs such as Levaquin, Floxin, and Noroxin. "If there is ever a group of drugs that has taken a beating, it is these," said UCSF pharmacy chief Guglielmo.

Against Acinetobacter—a bug responsible for rising numbers of bloodstream and lung infections in intensive care units, as well as among combat casualties in Iraq—Cipro's effectiveness fell from 80 percent in 1999 to 10 percent just four years later. Cipro has also lost ground against Pseudomonas aeruginosa, a common cause of pneumonia in hospitalized patients. Nearly 80 percent of the bugs tested were susceptible to Cipro in 1999. That fell to 65 percent by 2004.

At UCSF, doctors carefully monitor the trends in drug resistance and modify their prescribing patterns accordingly. As a result, they have been able to nudge some of these resistance levels down. Cipro's effectiveness against Acinetobacter crept up to 40 percent last year [2007], for example, but the overall trend remains alarming.

Although MRSA infections have been capturing headlines, bugs such as Acinetobacter, Klebsiella and Pseudomonas are keeping doctors awake at night. They come from a class of pathogens called Gram-negative bacteria, which typically have an extra layer of microbial skin to ward off antibiotics, and internal pumps that literally drive out antibiotics that penetrate.

Gram-negative infections have always been difficult to treat, and few new drugs are in development. Some researchers believe that the pipeline for new antibiotics is drying up because it is simply getting more difficult to outwit the bugs. "It may be that we've already found all the good antibiotics," warned Chambers, San Francisco General Hospital's infectious disease chief. "If that is so, then we've really got to be careful how we use the ones we have."

Some researchers believe that the pipeline for new antibiotics is drying up because it is simply getting more difficult to outwit the bugs.

Bacteria's Natural Evolution

Terry Hazen, senior scientist at Lawrence Berkeley National Laboratory and director of its ecology program, is not at all surprised by the tenacity of our bacterial foes. "We are talking about 3.5 billion years of evolution," he said. "They are the dominant life on Earth."

Bacteria have invaded virtually every ecological niche on the planet. Human explorers of extreme environments such as deep wells and mines are still finding new bacterial species. "As you go deeper into the subsurface, thousands and thousands of feet, you find bacteria that have been isolated for millions of years—and you find multiple antibiotic resistance," Hazen said.

In his view, when bacteria develop resistance to modern antibiotics, they are merely rolling out old tricks they mastered eons ago in their struggle to live in harsh environments in competition with similarly resilient species.

Drug industry economics are also a factor. "It takes a hell of a lot of effort to find the next really good drug," said Steven Projan, vice president of New Jersey pharmaceutical giant Wyeth Inc.

The costs of bringing a new drug to market are hotly debated. A Tufts University study estimated $802 million; the consumer group Public Citizen pegs it at $110 million. Either way, the investment is huge.

By 1990, according to the Infectious Diseases Society of America, half the major drugmakers in Japan and the United States had cut back or halted antibiotic research. Since 2000, some of the biggest names in pharmaceutical development— Roche, Bristol-Myers Squibb, Abbott Laboratories, Eli Lilly, Aventis and Procter & Gamble—had joined the exodus.

By common measures used to gauge the profit potential of new drugs, antibiotics fall way behind, Projan explained. For every $100 million that a new antibiotic might yield, after projected revenue and expenses are tallied, a new cancer drug will generate $300 million. A new drug for arthritis, by this same analysis, brings in $1.1 billion. Investors have been placing their bets accordingly.

In 2002, Wyeth had sharply curtailed its own antibiotic drug discovery programs. "We tried to get out of the field, but one of the reasons we did not get out altogether is we feel we have a public responsibility to fund more research," said Projan.

Wyeth's decision to keep some antibiotic research alive eventually paid off. In June 2005, the FDA licensed Tygacil, an intravenous antibiotic for complicated skin diseases such as drug-resistant staph infection. Only one new antibiotic for oral or intravenous use has won FDA approval since.

Pointing a Finger at Doctors

The waning of antibiotics in the arsenal of modern medicine has been going on for so long that some doctors fear a kind of complacency has set in. Increasingly, the medical profession is pointing a finger at itself.

"We have behaved very badly," said Dr. Louis Rice, a Harvard-educated, Columbia-trained specialist in infectious diseases. "We have made a lot of stupid choices."

His words brought a nervous silence to thousands of his colleagues, as he delivered a keynote speech in 2006 for the American Society for Microbiology's annual conference in San Francisco.

Rice, a professor at Cleveland's Case Western Reserve University, said doctors and drug companies alike are responsible for breeding resistance by "the indiscriminate dumping of antibiotics into our human patients."

Drug companies . . . have a responsibility to refill the nation's depleted medicine chest.

Drug-resistant germs contaminate the bedrails, the catheter lines, the blood pressure cuffs and even the unwashed hands of doctors, nurses and orderlies. The germs keep evolving, swapping drug-resistance traits with other microbes. He likened American intensive-care units—the high-tech enclaves where the most seriously ill patients are treated—to "toxic waste dumps."

Drug companies, he said, have a responsibility to refill the nation's depleted medicine chest. He suggested that a tax—similar to a Superfund tax placed on polluters to clean up toxic waste sites—be imposed on companies that have dropped antibiotic research. It would support drugmakers that are still in the game. "Your products that you've made billions and billions and billions and billions of dollars on have created this problem, and you can't just walk away," he said.

Rice has stressed that the existing arsenal of antibiotics should be used wisely, and that often means sparingly. During a half century of antibiotic use, he said, there is scant research on how short a course of drugs is actually needed to cure a patient. Instead, doctors routinely prescribe a week to 10-day course of drugs recommended by manufacturers. If patients are taking antibiotics after their infections are truly gone, they are creating conditions that breed resistance. Indeed, a Dutch study showed that one kind of pneumonia can be treated just as successfully with three days of amoxicillin as with the traditional eight.

Since drug companies cannot be expected to spend money on research that could trim sales of their products, federally funded agencies such as the National Institutes of Health should do the job, Rice said in a recent interview.

He also took his own specialty to task for failing to protect the most important weapons in its arsenal. Infectious disease experts at hospitals must find the "backbone" to stop other doctors from prescribing antibiotics unnecessarily, Rice said. He argued they should assert their authority to control antibiotic usage, just as cancer specialists have a say in which chemotherapy drugs are prescribed by surgeons.

And all health care professionals, he added, "have to wash their damn hands."

Drug Companies Promote the Overuse of Antibiotic Drugs

Joel Fuhrman, M.D.

Joel Fuhrman is a board-certified family physician who special-izes in preventing and reversing disease through nutritional and natural methods. His private practice is located in Flemington, New Jersey.

Antibiotic use has skyrocketed in recent years, but the mis-use of antibiotics isn't a new problem. Since the 1970s, medical studies have concluded that as much as 80 percent of all outpatient prescriptions are prescribed inappropriately.

The Role of Drug Companies

Antibiotic sales are soaring, but—in direct response—so are drug-resistant infections. As more and more antibiotics are used inappropriately, more and more strains of bacteria are mutating and becoming resistant to antibiotics. As a result, many patients who have infections that in the past could have been appropriately and effectively treated with antibiotics will die because the antibiotics will no longer work.

Drug companies are a big part of this problem. They pro-mote the use of their products through widespread advertising and the practice of giving free samples of the more potent, broad-spectrum antibiotics to doctors. The more widely these newer (and often ten times more expensive) antibiotics are used, the greater the chances that the bacteria will develop re-sistance.

Demanding Patients

Many patients don't think a doctor is doing his job if he doesn't prescribe antibiotics or other medication. If he doesn't

Joel Fuhrman, M.D., "Antibiotics for Colds, Bronchitis, and Sinusitis," www.DrFuhrman .com, January 2004. Reproduced by permission. www.DrFuhrman.com.

prescribe the medication they want, some patients actually will look for another doctor who will. For example, Robert Dristan is an emergency room physician well aware of the dangerous and inappropriate overuse of antibiotics. He told me that he sees a steady stream of patients with colds, bronchitis, or the flu. He always patiently describes the viral nature of these ailments, explains that no antibiotic can kill a virus, and informs patients that inappropriate use of antibiotics for these conditions could only harm them. He said that on more than one occasion, patients for whom he did not prescribe antibiotics returned, waving bottles of pills in his face, triumphantly stating, "My doctor said I almost had pneumonia." Patients can easily find a doctor willing to fabricate a diagnosis to justify coming to the rescue with a treatment.

Once a patient called me screaming on the telephone that her husband came to me for an antibiotic for his terrible cold, and all he got was a lecture. She wanted her money back and said she and her husband would never be coming again. Numerous patients have made similar demands. Most doctors perpetuate this problem because they give in to the pressure to prescribe antibiotics. They like to appear that they are offering an important and necessary service by writing prescriptions.

Antibiotics are the appropriate treatment for severe bacterial infections.

Powerful Medicine

Antibiotics are not harmless. Their use should not be undertaken without a convincing prognosis that serious harm will result if the antibiotic is not used. Antibiotics kill the normal bacteria that inhabit the intestines. These healthy bacteria serve an important function in digestion and production of fatty acids and nutrients. The use of antibiotics, and the change in flora that results, reduces vitamin absorption (for example, of vitamin K) and can lead to nutritional deficiency.

Furthermore, the use of antibiotics results in yeast overgrowth. It can cause severe allergic reaction, as well as food and environmental allergies to develop more readily. Overuse of antibiotics also can result in future infections with more serious (and resistant) bacterial organisms. Side effects can range from mild diarrhea and stomach upset to severe bone marrow suppression and serum sickness.

When to Use Antibiotics

Antibiotics are the appropriate treatment for severe bacterial infections. These infections include cellulitis, Lyme disease, pneumonia, joint infections, cat bites, meningitis, and bronchitis in a long-term smoker. Bronchitis in a non-smoker is just a bad cold. Almost every viral syndrome involves the bronchial tree and sinuses. The presence of yellow, brown, or green mucus does not indicate the need for an antibiotic. Likewise, sinusitis is not an appropriate diagnosis for the routine use of an antibiotic. Antibiotics should be reserved for the more serious sinus infections that show evidence of persistent symptoms lasting more than a week, such as continual fever and headache that accompanies facial pain and facial tenderness.

Childhood Ear Infections

Ear infections (otitis media) are the most common medical problem in children under seven years of age in the United States. Not only do nine out of ten children develop at least one ear infection each year, almost one-third of them develop chronic congestion with fluid in the middle ear that can lead to hearing loss and make the child a candidate for myringotomy or tube placement. Children who are breast fed for over a year have been shown to have many fewer infections than those weaned earlier. Studies also point to the fact that most ear infections early in life are viral, not bacterial. The vast majority of ear infections resolve nicely on their own, whether bacterial or viral, without an antibiotic. An international study following 3,660 children treated by general practitioners in nine countries showed that antibiotics did not improve the rate of recovery from ear infections.

It is common practice in this country to treat all ear infections with an antibiotic. Whether bacterial or not, our children get a routine prescription for an antibiotic at every minor illness. This cycle often is repeated many times, which may beget other medical problems in adulthood. This use of antibiotics early in life is likely a contributor to the increasing incidence of allergies and asthma and other problems later in life. Medical studies have linked a significant increased incidence of asthma, hay fever, and eczema to those who received multiple antibiotic prescriptions early in childhood, especially in the first year of life.

Conservative Treatment

In Europe, antibiotics are used for ear infections only when there is persistent drainage or persistent pain because these infections resolve on their own, without treatment, over 85 percent of the time. Studies show that the majority of ear infections are of viral etiology. For example, a microbiologic survey found that 75 percent of pediatric ear infections were caused by common respiratory viruses. Generally speaking, the use of antibiotics should be reserved for serious infections, not conditions the body is well equipped to resolve on its own. More and more physicians and authorities are recommending only treating ear infections with antibiotics when symptoms are not improving after three days and they are accompanied by drainage, fever, or persistent pain. Instead, ear drops for pain relief and other pain relievers can be used if the child is too uncomfortable to sleep.

A British study reported on 168 children treated in this manner. Antibiotics only were used if the illness followed an unusual course with high fever or profound weakness, or if the child had a history of purulent meningitis or a concurrent documented bacterial infection. They followed up on any child who did not recover in the typical time frame. As a result of this well-designed protocol, antibiotics were recommended by the physicians in only 10 children—fewer than 6 percent of all children presenting with acute ear infections. No serious complications, such as mastoiditis, meningitis, or permanent hearing loss, were observed.

This is similar to the way I treat childhood ear infections, except I also incorporate nutritional excellence, which I find reduces even further the likelihood of needing an antibiotic. The children of families who adopt my dietary recommendations simply stop getting ear infections.

Drug Companies Are Leading the Fight Against Resistant Infections

Billy Tauzin

Billy Tauzin is president and CEO of Pharmaceutical Research and Manufacturers of America (PhRMA), a trade group representing drug companies.

Infectious diseases have killed and crippled people throughout history. Until the 1920s, infectious diseases were the leading cause of death in the United States. Today, vaccines and antibiotics have proven to be effective treatments, but infectious diseases still pose a very serious threat to patients. Recently, some infectious pathogens, such as staphococcal, have become resistant to current treatments. Diseases once considered conquered, such as tuberculosis, have reemerged as a growing health threat. Other infectious agents have been manipulated for use in bioterrorist attacks.

As antibiotics have become less effective against Staphylocossus aureus—or staph—several potential vaccines are in development that would prevent [infection].

Antibiotic Research Continues

America's pharmaceutical researchers are developing 388 medicines and vaccines to combat humankind's oldest and most tenacious enemy—infectious diseases. Each of these medicines in development is either in human clinical trials or awaiting Food and Drug Administration approval.

Among the medicines now being tested are 83 antibiotics/ antibacterials, 75 antivirals for treating such viruses as hepatitis, herpes and influenza; and 146 vaccines to prevent diseases from staph infections to pneumococcal infections. Not included in this report are medicines in development for HIV infection. A 2006 survey by PhRMA [Pharmaceutical Research and Manufacturers of America] found 77 medicines and vaccines in testing for HIV/AIDS and AIDS-related conditions.

Some examples of the potential medicines for fighting infectious diseases include:

- A first-in-class medicine designed specifically to inhibit drug-resistant strains of *Staphylococcus aureus*.

- A medicine for the treatment of hepatitis C that is part of a new class of drugs to regulate innate immunity. It is believed the new medicine interacts with a specific receptor that is present on certain immune system cells.

- A vaccine adjuvant that can enhance biowarfare vaccines by resulting in fewer shots and faster immunity.

- A medicine that stops the life cycle of the bacterium that causes tuberculosis.

- As antibiotics have become less effective against *Staphylococcus aureus*—or staph—several potential vaccines are in development that would prevent patients from ever being infected in the first place.

Pharmaceutical researchers also are focusing their efforts on new treatments for fungal infections, herpes, influenza, malaria, meningitis, pneumonia, respiratory infections, rotavirus, sepsis, smallpox, and urinary tract infections, among others.

Infectious diseases will never be wiped out. But new knowledge, new technologies, and a huge commitment of resources by both the government and America's pharmaceutical research companies can help meet the continuing—and ever-changing—threat from infectious diseases.

Drug Companies Have Few Financial Incentives to Produce Antibacterial Drugs

Paul Gigot

Paul Gigot is the editorial page editor and vice president of The Wall Street Journal, *a well-known U.S.-based business and financial newspaper.*

This week on "The Journal Editorial Report," attack of the superbug. It's the season's most sensational story, but how serious a public health threat are infections like MRSA [methicillin-resistant Staphylococcus aureus]?. . .

Paul Gigot: Welcome to "The Journal Editorial Report." I'm Paul Gigot. Well, it's this season's equivalent of shark attacks: almost daily reports of new cases of a virulent and drug-resistant bacteria known as MRSA. A practicing physician, Dr. Scott Gottlieb recently left the No. 2 spot at the Food and Drug Administration [FDA]. Earlier, I asked him how serious this public health threat this so-called superbug really is.

Scott Gottlieb: Well, it is a serious problem. It's not a new problem. This has been a problem that's been ongoing for years now where we've been seeing more and more of these resistant infections, particularly in the hospital. Doctors have been confronting hospitalized patients that have these very complicated infections that are resistant to a lot of our traditional drugs.

What's changing is that we're seeing more and more patients come in from the community with seemingly ordinary infections—urinary tract infections, pneumonia, bronchitis, even skin infections—that are complicated or caused by these very resistant pathogens. And that's a big concern to patients; it's a big concern to doctors, because your first instinct is to use the ordinary antibiotic to treat these patients. And then you find out three or four days later when the infection progresses and becomes, in some cases, life-threatening that it's complicated with one of these vicious new pathogens.

But we've read about some of these very high-profile cases, scary cases, of young kids brought in off the street with a seemingly mild malady, and then somehow they get this terribly virulent, fatal infection. But in terms of mortality, overall, across the entire United States, compared to heart disease or cancer, the really big killers, how serious is this? Where does this fit in?

It's unclear. The statistics on this are hard to ascertain. There was a study done recently by the CDC [Centers for Disease Control and Prevention, the nation's top health agency] which tried to estimate the prevalence of MRSA by calculating an estimate off of data they collected in about six hospitals. I'm not sure how reliable that is. It's fairly significant. A lot of people in the hospitals and even the community who succumb to their illnesses succumb because of infections.

We don't have a lot of new antibiotics coming along that are fundamentally different enough to attack some of these very resistant pathogens.

We're talking tens of thousands of fatalities?

We're talking at least tens of thousands, absolutely, from hospital-acquired infections and serious infections. But the *New England Journal [of Medicine]* reported about four or five years ago on the rising incidence of these community-acquired infections being with resistant pathogens. That's really what's new. That's the scary part.

OK, now, you wrote in a newspaper I like, The Wall Street Journal, *recently, the following: "As we make progress in fields like cancer, we are taking a U-turn on bacteria." How so?*

That's right. Because a lot of the drugs that we've gotten used to using, the mainstay drugs, are now not effective against a lot of these resistant pathogens. The bugs have learned how to outsmart the drugs. And when you look at the pipeline of new drugs that are in development, we don't have a lot of new antibiotics coming along that are fundamentally different enough to attack some of these very resistant pathogens. And that's because a lot of the companies that invested in this space 20, 15 years ago have gotten out of it. Abbott and Lilly, which were some of the pioneers in antibiotic drug development, have gotten out entirely.

Why have they gotten out of it? The figures you cited, it was 13—only 13 new antibiotics under development in the big drug companies now, compared to 60, 10 years ago. That's a really startling statistic. What's the problem for these drug companies?

Only 13 new antibiotics [are] under development in the big drug companies now, compared to 60, 10 years ago.

Right. Now, there's a lot of innovation going on in the biotech companies so that—

The smaller entrepreneurs?

Right, the smaller—which sometimes have more obstacles bringing the drugs to market. But it's a complicated problem. Part of it is that the market for these drugs isn't that attractive. It's not that lucrative, so the incentives aren't there. Part of it is that if you do develop a very effective antibiotic, hospitals, doctors, public health agencies are going to try to restrict the use of that drug, try to hold it in reserve.

The market for these [antibiotic] drugs isn't that attractive. It's not that lucrative, so the incentives aren't there.

But that's smart. You need to do that, right?

Right. But it also reduces the potential market and so makes the compensation structure very complicated. And part of it is regulatory. It's not so much the FDA set a high bar to the approval of these drugs, although in some cases it has. But the FDA has been changing the regulatory requirements, and the one thing companies hate is regulatory uncertainty. And in fact, there have been at least two companies recently that did what FDA told them to do three years ago, got their drugs to the point of submitting it to the agency, and the agency said, Well, it works according to what we told you to do, but we've changed our requirements.

The FDA has been changing the regulatory requirements, and the one thing companies hate is regulatory uncertainty.

Yeah, but I could see some of our viewers saying, OK, now look, hey, there we go again. The big drug companies, big pharma, all they care about is profits. They don't care about these small drugs, and that's why we don't have these antibiotics. Is that really a problem, that they're just so profit-driven that that's all they care about?

I think it's a problem that these take significant investments, and if you know you're not going to get a return on that investment, it makes it hard to justify putting that money in.

How do you change the incentives?

The drug companies have derisked themselves. A lot of the risk-taking now is in the smaller biotech companies, no question about that. But I think from a policy standpoint, there are things you can do to try to create incentives around developing the drugs that treat these superinfections. So we look at things like the Orphan Drug Act, which tried to incentivize—

—1983, which tried to give special patent protections and other things to drugs that treat rare diseases.

Right.

Should antibiotics be treated under the Orphan Drug Act?

I think when you're talking about developing a drug to treat the superinfections, where you know, from a policy standpoint, if the company's successful you're going to restrict use of the drug because you want to hold it in reserve, I think we should think about offering policy incentives to do that, because the policy environment is intruding upon the potential market for the drug. I think the policy environment needs to try to come up with a solution to incentivize that kind of development.

You worked at the FDA. You've been around Washington. Is this going to take—before Congress and the bureaucracy start to change these incentives, are we going to have to have some really widespread mortality and a bigger problem with these kinds of infections?

Good question. Hard to say. I think the attention around MRSA has definitely woken up some policy makers. I compare this to the shark attacks. This is a problem that's been going on for four or five years. Suddenly, Matt Lauer [co-host of NBC's *Today* Show] discovered it on TV. So—

But shark attacks, there are only about two or three fatalities a year. This is really a lot bigger.

No, that's right. There's actually activity on [Capitol] Hill right now, looking at legislation to try to incentivize this kind of development. I think that what's been proposed so far isn't on target. It's trying to incentivize the wrong kind of drug development, if you will. But I think policy makers do get it, and they are moving in the direction of trying to address this issue. Whether or not they're able to do it in the near term or it's going to take another round of media to push them in the direction, I'm not sure. It is bipartisan, which is interesting. You're seeing Democrats talk about incentives for drug companies to do this kind of development.

All right, well, thanks for watching this and pushing it. We'll be watching.

Smaller Drug Companies Are Still Doing Antibiotic Research

Andriy Luzhetskyy, Stefan Pelzer, and Andreas Bechthold

Andriy Luzhetskyy, Stefan Pelzer, and Andreas Bechthold are medical researchers working in Germany.

One reason for the current crisis in antibiotic development is the low return on investment, which is intrinsic to anti-infective drug development. Despite this, smaller pharmaceutical companies are attempting to address the medical need for new antibiotics. Natural products have played a major role in antibiotic drug discovery since 1941 when penicillin was introduced to the market, and currently natural products are again the most important source for promising drug candidates. . . .

The Abandonment of Antibiotic Research

More than 60% of the 877 small-molecule NCEs [novel chemical entries, referring to drugs that contain no elements that have been approved by the U.S. Food and Drug Administration] and 79% of all small-molecule antibacterials introduced as drugs worldwide between 1981 and 2002 can be traced to natural products. The reasons for the success of natural products are their great structural diversity and the fact that evolution over millions of years preselected these compounds for interaction and activity. The dominance and pharmaceutical success of natural products is most obvious in the field of antibiotics. It is surprising that the > [more than] 200 antibacterial drugs, which have been launched for human therapy since the invention of the sulfonamides by Domagk in

Andriy Luzhetskyy, Stefan Pelzer, and Andreas Bechthold, "The Future of Natural Products as a Source of New Antibiotics," *Current Opinion in Investigational Drugs*, vol. 8, 2007, pp. 608–613. Copyright © 2007 Thomson Reuters. All rights reserved. Reproduced by permission.

1935, belong to a limited number of antibacterial classes. From 11 antibacterial classes introduced for systemic use in humans, 8 are derived from natural products.

Antibacterial research was abandoned because of the belief that there was no real need for new antibiotics, and for economic reasons.

Despite the overall success of natural products and the fact that antibiotics have saved millions of lives, two trends have been observed, particularly in large pharmaceutical companies, during the last decade: the downsizing or even termination of both natural product and antibiotic research. Reasons for the decline of natural product research include the following: (i) traditional extract-based screening leads to the re-discovery of previously known compounds; (ii) structural complexity of natural products renders chemical total synthesis and derivatization more difficult; (iii) because of supply problems, the time required to develop a natural product from an extract hit to a pharmaceutical drug is long; and (iv) a focus on combinatorial chemistry to generate huge compound libraries is needed to fullfil the demand of HTS [high-throughput screening, a scientific experimentation method especially used in drug discovery] technologies.

Antibacterial research was abandoned because of the belief that there was no real need for new antibiotics, and for economic reasons such as the pressure of generic antibacterial drugs as well as the shift toward the development of drugs for the treatment of chronic diseases which appears commercially more attractive. This is despite the fact that antibiotics are the third largest pharmaceutical drug market segment with more than US $25.7 billion global sales in 2004. However, there are several reasons underlying the urgent need for new antibiotics: (i) currently, infectious diseases are still the second major cause of death worldwide; (ii) the emergence and spread of multiresistant pathogens particularly in the hospital environment; and (iii) the constant decrease in the total number of antibacterial agents that have been approved by the FDA [U.S. Food and Drug Administration].

Recently, researchers in the field of antibiotic development have started to develop new strategies and new technologies which hopefully will help to overcome the antibiotic crisis.

Small Companies Doing Research

There are several excellent reviews analyzing the status of the current clinical development pipelines of antibacterial agents. According to these reports, between 15 and 20 small-molecule antibacterials intended for systemic use are undergoing phase I clinical trials or beyond. With the exception of several novel quinolones, an oxazolidinone and a diaminopyridine [all types of antibiotics], the majority of these compounds are natural products or natural-product derivatives. These include novel derivatives of existing antibiotic classes such as the β-lactams, a cephalosporin that is currently at the pre-registration stage of development; faropenem daloxate, a penem undergoing phase III clinical trials; ceftaroline fosamil, a cephalosporin in phase III trials; and tomopenem, a carbapenem in phase II trials; the macrolides/ketolides, in phase III trials; glycopeptides, filed for FDA approval; telavancin in pre-registration; and oritavancin, streptogramins, tetracyclines ansamycin. . . .

Several small pharmaceutical companies and biotech companies . . . licensed antibacterial compounds from large pharmaceuticals companies after development had been terminated.

After examination of the current drug development pipelines, two important aspects should be highlighted: (i) an oral pleuromutilin derivative, acting on protein biosynthesis and currently in phase I clinical evaluation, is the only remaining representative of a chemical scaffold not previously found in marketed drugs for clinical systemic use . . . and (ii) large pharmaceutical companies are no longer considered the main driver of antibiotic development. However, several small pharmaceutical companies and biotech companies, such as Cubist Pharmaceuticals Inc and Oscient Pharmaceuticals Corp licensed antibacterial compounds from large pharmaceutical companies after development had been terminated. The development of daptomycin, the first lipopeptide antibiotic to reach market in 2004, is the first case study of a biotech company that successfully developed an antibacterial drug, which had been outlicensed by Eli Lilly & Co after its discontinuation of phase II studies owing to adverse events.

Friulimicin B was originally discovered by the former Hoechst Marion Roussel and is now under investigation by Combinature Biopharm AG. A phase I clinical trial of friulimicin B was initiated in Switzerland in June 2007. While the lipopeptide antibiotic friulimicin is, from a chemical point of view, similar to the lipodepsipeptide daptomycin, it is the first member of a novel class of bactericidal lipopeptide antibiotics. In contrast to the membrane-interfering daptomycin, friulimicin appears to target late-stage cell wall synthesis by inhibiting the biosynthesis of the lipid I precursor, as has been shown for the structurally related antibiotic amphomycin. Because of this unique and new mechanism, friulimicin can be considered a novel class of lipopeptide antibiotics.

Thus, only a few compounds (eg, pleuromutilin and friulimicin) represent novel classes addressing novel bacterial targets and therefore further novel classes are urgently needed to combat multiresistant Gram-positive and the emerging multiresistant Gram-negative pathogens such as *Acinetobacter, Pseudomonas* and diverse *Enterobacteriaceae*.

Many Antibiotics Still to Be Discovered from Natural Sources

For more than 60 years actinomycetes [bacteria that live in the soil] and fungi have been the most fruitful groups of organisms in antibiotic production and will likely remain the main source for new antibiotics in the future. Mathematical models ... estimated that more than 10^5 antibiotics are produced by streptomycetes [a type of actinomycete] and only a small portion (3%) of these antibiotics have been discovered thus far. To find the remaining antibiotics will require new approaches and technologies. ...

Drug discovery companies [however,] often try to avoid dealing with natural products because their complex structures represent a challenge for ... medicinal chemists. Developments in the manipulation of structures of complex bacterial natural products via genetic engineering have helped to overcome this problem. ...

Although some novel compounds are under investigation, there is still an urgent unmet medical need for the development of novel antibacterial classes, and microbial natural products still appear as the most promising source for drug identification. Innovative technologies, such as high-throughput miniaturized screening of uncommon actinomycetes, genome sequencing and genome mining, and combinatorial biosynthesis will strongly support antibiotic development in the next decade.

CHAPTER 4

How Can the Problem of Resistant Infections Be Remedied?

Chapter Preface

Many health experts criticize the U.S. government for failing to take concrete action to address the growing challenge of resistant infections. The federal government's main response has been the creation of the U.S. Interagency Task Force on Antimicrobial Resistance, which aims to develop a national plan to combat antimicrobial resistance. The Task Force, created in 1999, is chaired by the U.S. Food and Drug Administration (FDA), the Centers for Disease Control and Prevention (CDC), and the National Institutes of Health (NIH)—three of the nation's top health agencies. Seven other federal agencies make up the rest of the Task Force.

In 2001, after consulting with a wide range of interested groups and the public, the Task Force published the "Public Health Action Plan to Combat Antimicrobial Resistance"—a blueprint that laid out specific federal actions to address the emerging threat of antibiotic resistance. The Action Plan was divided into four areas: surveillance, prevention and control, research, and product development. The surveillance part of the plan emphasized collecting information and statistics about the emergence and spread of resistant bacteria and the use of antibiotic drugs. The prevention and control aspect of the plan was aimed at controlling both the medical and agricultural use of antibiotic drugs to prolong the effectiveness of existing antibiotics. The research goals of the Action Plan were to encourage and expand existing research in antibiotic resistance to improve treatment of resistant infections. In the area of product development, the plan sought to stimulate the development of new antibiotic drugs and vaccines by creating market incentives for the pharmaceutical industry.

Unfortunately, the Task Force was never fully funded, and the federal agencies that make up the body have been unable to effectively implement the four main elements of the Action

Plan. In 2003 the FDA and the CDC launched a campaign—called *Get Smart: Know When Antibiotics Work*—aimed at educating consumers and health care professionals on the appropriate use of antibiotics. As part of the campaign, the CDC developed clinical guidelines to educate health professionals about the best ways to use antimicrobials, and the FDA issued labeling regulations for the appropriate use of systemic antibacterial drugs in humans. In addition, the FDA, the NIH, and the Agency for Healthcare Research and Quality (AHRQ) have funded or supported a few research and clinical studies directed at diagnosing resistant infections, using antibiotics, and developing vaccines. Since 2001, however, no further major actions have been taken or proposed by the federal government to stimulate research and development of antibiotics or vaccines.

The Task Force is now working to update the Action Plan for the next five years. In December 2007, the Task Force held a meeting of more than fifty consultants from the United States and around the world to solicit input and recommendations for a new plan. The consultants included health experts from both human and veterinary medicine, pharmaceutical companies, agriculture interests, clinical microbiology, epidemiology, infectious disease and infection control specialists, and state and local public health departments. The meeting also was attended by representatives of federal agencies and was open to the public. Based on the comments received, a revised Action Plan has been drafted around five focus areas: reducing inappropriate antimicrobial use; reducing the spread of antibiotic resistant microorganisms; enhancing laboratory capacity to detect resistant microorganisms; encouraging the development of new anti-infective products, vaccines, and other therapies; and supporting basic research on antibiotic resistance.

The federal legislature has been similarly slow to react to the resistant infections crisis. Several pieces of legislation were introduced in the 109th Congress—spanning the period from January 2005 to January 2007—but none of these bills were enacted. In 2007, however, the Congress passed the Food and Drug Administration Amendments Act of 2007, legislation that included provisions to enable the government to gather data about the extent of the spread of antibiotic resistance. Among other provisions, for example, the law requires the U.S. Government Accountability Office (GAO) to study the causes of infections that occur in hospitals and to evaluate hospital infection-control procedures.

Another bill, the Strategies to Address Antimicrobial Resistance Act (STAAR), also was introduced in both houses of Congress in 2007. This legislation sought to create an Office of Antimicrobial Resistance in the U.S. Department of Health and Human Services (HHS) and a Public Health Antimicrobial Advisory Board. The goal of the bill was to develop a coordinated federal effort to combat antibiotic-resistant infection, an effort that would begin by gathering data about resistant infections and their spread. The STAAR legislation, however, was never passed by Congress. Other bills (S.2351 and H.R.4200) introduced into the Senate and House in 2007—to provide tax credits for the research and development of critically needed antibiotic and antiviral drugs, vaccines, and other products—also failed to pass.

Much of such proposed legislation was widely supported by health experts and organizations. In addition to efforts to keep track of the spread of antibiotic-resistant diseases and to promote more prudent use of existing antibiotics, many health experts stress that the government must encourage drug companies to reinvest in research and development of antibiotics, vaccines, and other therapies that might combat the resistant disease crisis. The viewpoints in this chapter provide an overview of this and other proposals for remedying the resistant infection problem.

The Nontherapeutic Use of Antibiotics in Food Animal Production Should Be Banned

Jay P. Graham

Jay P. Graham is a consultant to the Pew Commission on Industrial Farm Animal Production and a research fellow for the Johns Hopkins Bloomberg School of Public Health.

Antimicrobials are a critical defense in the fight against infectious bacteria that can cause disease and death in humans. Their value as a resource in human medicine is being squandered through inappropriate use in animals raised for food. The method that now predominates in food animal agriculture—applying constant low doses of antimicrobials to billions of animals—facilitates the rapid emergence of resistant disease-causing bacteria and compromises the ability of medicine to treat disease, making it clear that such inappropriate and indiscriminate use must end.

Antibiotics in Agriculture

A wide range of antimicrobial drugs are permitted for use in food animal production in the U.S. These drugs represent most of the major classes of clinically important antimicrobials, from penicillin to third-generation cephalosporin compounds. In some cases, new drugs were licensed for agricultural use in advance of approvals for clinical use. In the case of quinupristin-dalfopristin—an analog of virginiamycin, which is used in food animal production—this decision by the FDA [U.S. Food and Drug Administration] resulted in the emergence of resistance in human isolates prior to eventual

Jay P. Graham, "Statement of Jay P. Graham before the U.S. Senate Committee on Health, Education, Labor, and Pensions," *Pew Commission on Industrial Farm Animal Production*, www.ncifap.org, June 24, 2008. Reproduced by permission.

clinical registration, thus demonstrating how feed additive use can compromise the potential utility of a new tool in fighting infectious disease in humans. Agricultural use can also significantly shorten the "useful life" of existing antimicrobials for combating human or animal disease.

While discussion of the issue of declining effectiveness of antimicrobials often centers on the importance of ensuring the proper use of antimicrobials in human medicine, the fact is that most antimicrobials used in the U.S. are used as "growth promoters" in food animal production, not human medicine. In North Carolina alone, the use of antimicrobials as a feed supplement has been estimated to exceed all U.S. antimicrobial use in human medicine. A relatively small percentage of antimicrobial use in food animal production is to treat sick animals, and much of what is needed for therapeutic purposes is the direct result of the animal husbandry practices of crowding large numbers of food animals in small confined spaces, thereby increasing the chance that diseases will spread through food animal populations.

From a public health perspective, it clearly makes good sense to remove antimicrobials for growth promotion in food animal production.

Exposure of bacteria to sub-lethal concentrations of antimicrobial agents is particularly effective in driving the selection of resistant strains, and under conditions of constant antimicrobial use, resistant strains are advantaged in terms of reproduction and spread. Because of the rapidity of bacterial reproduction, these changes can be expressed with great efficiency.

Exacerbating the problem of using antimicrobials for growth promotion of food animals is the fact that bacteria can share genetic material that encodes resistance to antimicrobials. It is estimated that transferable resistance genes ac-

143

count for more than 95% of antibiotic resistance. These events have been frequently detected in resistant *E. coli* isolated from consumer meat products. At this point, most research has focused on specific patterns of resistance in selected disease-causing organisms—a "one bug, one drug" definition of the problem. But this discounts the fact that it is the community of genetic resources that determines the rate and propagation of resistance.

From a public health perspective, it clearly makes good sense to remove antimicrobials for growth promotion in food animal production. When this is done, resistance in disease-causing organisms tends to decrease significantly. Studies carried out in Europe have demonstrated a rapid decrease in the prevalence of antimicrobial resistant *Enterococcus faecium* recovered from pigs and broilers after antimicrobials were removed. The prevalence of resistant enterococci isolates from human subjects also declined in the European Union (EU) over the same period.

Recent studies call into question the assumed economic benefits of using antimicrobials in animal feeds.

Addressing other animal agriculture practices, such as more thorough and frequent cleaning of animal feeding operation facilities, may also be needed in conjunction with cessation of using antimicrobials to eliminate reservoirs of antibiotic resistance bacteria from farms.

Recent studies call into question the assumed economic benefits of using antimicrobials in animal feeds. Historically, economic gains from using antimicrobials to promote growth have been thought to justify the expense of the drugs. Two recent large-scale studies—one with poultry and one with swine—found that the actual economic benefits were miniscule to nonexistent, and that the same financial benefits could instead be achieved by improving the management of the animals (e.g., cleaning out poultry houses). Even when improvements from growth promoting antimicrobials have been observed, their benefits are completely offset if costs from increased resistance are considered: loss of disease treatment options in humans and animals, increased health care costs, and more severe and enduring infections. These costs are usually "externalized" to the larger society and not captured in the price of the meat and poultry sold to consumers.

The Link Between Agriculture and Human Infections

There are industry trade groups that argue that using antimicrobials in the food animal production process does not pose a threat to public health. But, numerous studies support a strong link between the introduction of an antimicrobial into animal feeds and increased resistance in disease-causing organisms isolated from humans. Resistant disease-causing organisms can affect the public through food routes and environmental routes.

Food routes: In the U.S., antimicrobial resistant disease-causing organisms are highly prevalent in meat and poultry products, including disease-causing organisms in meats that are resistant to the broad-spectrum antimicrobials penicillin, tetracycline and erythromycin. Animals given antimicrobials in their feed contain a higher prevalence of multidrug-resistant *E. coli* than animals produced on farms where they are not exposed to antibiotics, and the same disparity shows up when one compares the meat and poultry products consumers purchase from these two styles of production.

Environmental routes: Waste disposal is the major source of antimicrobial resistant disease causing organisms entering the environment from animal feeding operations. Each year, confined food animals produce an estimated 335 million tons of waste, which is deposited on land and enters water sources. This amount is more than 40 times the mass of human biosolids generated by publicly owned treatment works (7.6 million dry tons in 2005). No treatment requirements exist in the U.S. for animal waste before it is disposed of, usually on croplands—even though levels of antimicrobial resistant bacteria are present at high levels.

Antimicrobial resistant *E. coli* and resistance genes have been detected in groundwater sources for drinking water sampled near hog farms in North Carolina, Maryland, and Iowa. Groundwater provides drinking water for more than 97% of rural U.S. populations. In addition, antibiotics used in food animal production are regularly found in surface waters at low levels.

Resistant disease-causing organisms can also travel through the air from animal feeding operation facilities. At swine facilities using ventilation systems, resistant disease-causing organisms in the air have been detected as far away as 30 meters upwind and 150 meters downwind.

Farm workers and people living near animal feeding operations are at greatest risk for suffering the adverse effects of antimicrobial use in agriculture. Studies have documented their elevated risk of carrying antibiotic-resistant disease-causing organisms.

A Threat to Public Health

The rise of antimicrobial resistance in bacteria, in response to exposure to antimicrobial agents, is inevitable as all uses of antimicrobial agents drives the selection of resistant strains. Thus, there is the potential to lose this valuable resource in human medicine, which might well be finite and nonrenewable—once a disease-causing organism develops resistance to an antimicrobial, it may not be possible to restore its effectiveness. Declining antimicrobial effectiveness can be equated with resource extraction. The very notion of antimicrobial effectiveness as a natural resource is a new concept, so it is not surprising that there has been very little public discussion about the ethical implications of depleting this resource for non-essential purposes, such as for growth promotion in food animal production.

In 2003, the American Public Health Association (APHA), in its policy statement, said "the emerging scientific consensus is that antibiotics given to food animals contribute to antibiotic resistance transmitted to humans." APHA, the world's largest public health organization, also remarked that "an estimated 25–75 percent of feed antibiotics pass unchanged into manure waste."

Prudent public health policy . . . indicates that nontherapeutic uses of antimicrobials in food animal production should be ended.

For its part, the World Health Organization (WHO) has recommended that "in the absence of a public health safety evaluation, [governments should] terminate or rapidly phase out the use of antimicrobials for growth promotion if they are also used for treatment of humans."

For an industry that has become accustomed to using antimicrobials as growth promoters, the idea of stopping this practice might seem daunting. But, consider the case of Denmark, which in 1999 banned the use of antimicrobials as growth promoters. In 2002, the World Health Organization reported that:

". . . the termination of antimicrobial growth promoters in Denmark has dramatically reduced the food animal reservoir of enterococci resistant to these growth promoters, and therefore reduced a reservoir of genetic determinants (resistance genes) that encode antimicrobial resistance to several clinically important antimicrobial agents in humans."

The World Health Organization also reported there were no significant differences in the health of the animals or the bottom line of the producers. The European Union has followed suit with a ban on growth promoters that took effect in 2006.

Finally, prudent public health policy thus indicates that nontherapeutic uses of antimicrobials in food animal production should be ended. Economic analyses demonstrate that there is little economic benefit from using antimicrobials as feed additives, and that equivalent improvements in growth and feed consumption can be achieved by improved hygiene.

Policies Must Be Implemented to Prolong the Effectiveness of Antibiotic Drugs

Gary Feuerberg

Gary Feuerberg is a Washington, D.C., staff writer for Epoch Times, *an independent news media company based in New York.*

Modern medicine is rapidly approaching a crisis state. The antibiotics that we have depended upon for 65 years are losing their effectiveness, and death from drug-resistant pathogens are increasing in frequency.

"More than 63,000 patients in the United States die every year from hospital-acquired bacterial infections that are resistant to at least one common antibiotic . . ." says a new report released March 22 [2007], "Extending the Cure: Policy Responses to the Growing Threat of Antibiotic Resistance."

The research was conducted by Resources for the Future (RFF), a nonpartisan organization that conducts research in public health issues. This number is more deaths than from either AIDS, traffic accidents, or influenza. And the actual number is probably higher because many deaths attributed to other causes, may be really due to antibiotic-resistant infections.

In 1941 penicillin was first introduced, and since then the medical system has increasingly relied on antibiotics to control infectious diseases. Moreover, the successes of new procedures, such as kidney and heart transplants, as well as chemotherapy and surgery, were made possible by the crucial role that antibiotics play in preventing surgical site infections and saving the lives of patients with weakened immune systems.

Treating Resistant Infections

The best example of this problem of antibiotic resistance is the case of *Staphylococcus aureus (S. aureus)*, better known to lay people as "Staph" infection. Its mortality rate was reputed to be as high as 82% in the days before antibiotics. Then the "wonder" drug, penicillin, was introduced in 1941 and saved many lives and limbs from amputation during World War II.

However, resistance to penicillin emerged, and people began to die again from this infection. So, in 1960, penicillin was replaced with methicillin, which was effective against the penicillin resistant *S. aureus*. But by the 1970s, unfortunately, a methicillin-resistant *S. aureus* (MRSA) had evolved just as had happened to penicillin.

In 1974, only 2.4% of patients in U.S. hospitals with the "Staph" infection failed to respond to methicillin, the penicillin replacement, according to Ramanan Laxminarayan, Ph.D., who is a senior researcher at RFF and one of the primary authors of the report.

> *The problem is that each of the main players in our health care system ... has an interest ... which lead[s] to actions that are detrimental to the common good of all.*

Dr. Laxminarayan cites data that says that the MRSA prevalence increased to 29% in 1991, and to nearly 60% by 2003. The latter data is from the Centers for Disease Control and Prevention (CDC). MRSA prevalence rates in U.S. hospitals have grown more than 12% per year.

Note that even though methicillin—the "M" in "MRSA"—was found ineffective long ago and has been replaced, "MRSA" is still retained by the health professionals as the acronym used for the general phenomena of resistant *S. aureus* to a penicillin derived antibiotics.

The latest and possibly the last drug that can treat MRSA infections is vancomycin. But its massive use has given rise to vancomycin-resistant enterococci (VRE) and strains of MRSA resistant to vancomycin, according to Dr. Laxminarayan. The U.S. VRE rate of 12.6% is one of the highest in the world.

Drugs like penicillin and methicillin were inexpensive. Penicillin cost pennies a dose, but the most recent antibiotics "can run as high as a few thousand dollars for a course of treatment," says Dr. Laxminarayan. The chief reason for this huge expense is that the newer drugs are under patent. As our medical system has to rely more on very expensive treatments, this will have a profound effect on the poor and uninsured.

Moreover, patients typically have to be treated with two or more drugs to ensure the treatment will be successful. This is certainly an incentive to use multiple drugs rather than take a chance on a sequential drug treatment and jeopardize a patient's life.

New Policies for "Extending the Cure"

"Extending the Cure" addresses the problem of antibiotic resistance, not by trying to eliminate it which the report says is impossible. Instead, it assesses the pros and cons of various policies designed to protect antibiotic effectiveness by (1) delaying the emergence of resistant bacteria and (2) controlling better the spreading of the antibiotic-resistant bacteria.

The problem is that each of the main players in our health care system—health care providers, consumers, insurers, and pharmaceutical manufacturers—has an interest, such as maximizing company profits, avoiding lawsuits, or fighting off a life-threatening infection, which lead to actions that are detrimental to the common good of all. The report considers new incentives that hopefully will have as an outcome, the keeping of the antibiotic drugs effective as long as possible.

One set of policies that the report would like to put in place involves reducing antibiotic prescribing. Every time antibiotics are used, the "effective lifespan of that antibiotic and perhaps related drugs has been shortened," says the report.

Another way to reduce the need for antibiotics is to reduce transmissions in the hospital settings.

The United States has one of the highest rates of antibiotic prescribing in the world. Educating physicians and patients can help here, but reducing prescribing is an instance of choosing between the good of the individual versus society.

The need for antibiotics can sometimes be reduced by community vaccination campaigns. Presumably then there would be less sickness and fewer number of infections. The report suggests a national requirement for childhood pneumococcal vaccinations, which "could greatly reduce the need for antibiotics in children under the age of five, who consume a significant proportion of antibiotics used in the community," says the report.

Another way to reduce the need for antibiotics is to reduce transmissions in the hospital settings. Some methods discussed in the report are doing a better job in isolating patients who have the beginnings of a resistant infection, restricting the nursing staff with access to patients with such infections, and more rigorous attention to hand-washing and changing of caps and gowns.

The Netherlands stands out in Europe as a country with stricter controls of their MRSA infected patients—isolating the patients in private rooms and taking care not to infect other hospitals—and the result has been an extremely low rate of MRSA infections.

The Dutch, known for their war strategy of "search and destroy," are especially vigilant in controlling their MRSA problem. Patients from foreign hospitals and suspected MRSA carriers are screened and isolated, according to the *Eurosurveillance Monthly* (Mar 2000).

The Dutch form ad hoc MRSA teams to control the problem, and the board of directors, medical specialists, nurses, and other health care workers of the hospital may be required to cooperate with additional measures, including closure of wards. As a result, the above source states, "older antibiotics continue to be first line drugs in the treatment of serious infections."

However, it is difficult to persuade U.S. hospitals to the above actions when the use of antibiotics is less expensive. Moreover, the costs of staff time and other expenses related to infection control are borne by the hospital, while antibiotics are paid by health insurers.

Also, many patients use more than one hospital and so if one enlightened hospital makes the investment for better controls, it could result in a waste because the other area hospitals are not doing the same. In the Netherlands all the hospitals share the costs and benefits of superior infection control.

Hospitals Must Carefully Manage Their Antibiotic Prescriptions

Laura Landro

Laura Landro writes "The Informed Patient" column for The Wall Street Journal, *a leading U.S.-based financial and business newspaper.*

Hospitals are turning to a new breed of antibiotic SWAT team to win the war against "superbugs"—the bacteria that are outmaneuvering nearly every weapon in the arsenal of drugs long used to fight them.

The efforts, known as antimicrobial stewardship programs, team top pharmacists, infectious-disease specialists and microbiologists. The groups monitor the use of a hospital's antibiotics and restrict prescriptions of specific drugs when they become less effective at fighting infections. The heightened vigilance comes as the federal Medicare program plans to begin refusing to pay hospitals to treat preventable infections that patients contract while under the facilities' care.

Reducing the Use of Antibiotics

Some two million people acquire bacterial infections in U.S. hospitals each year, and 90,000 of those patients die as a result. Although antibiotics generally kill or inhibit the growth of susceptible bacteria, they also allow some bugs to survive and become resistant to the drugs. The current epidemic of MRSA [methicillin-resistant *Staphylococcus aureus*]—a form of drug-resistant staph found in hospitals and places such as school locker rooms—is just one example of the growing number of bacteria that have developed resistance to common drugs.

The aim is to get doctors to use the narrowest-spectrum antibiotic possible.

Now, two of the leading hospital purchasing groups are mounting new campaigns to reduce the use of antibiotics. VHA Inc., an alliance of more than 1,400 nonprofit hospitals, has launched a "Bugs and Drugs" program to help member institutions identify and manage resistance to antibiotics. Premier Inc., which represents more than 2,000 hospitals, is urging members to adopt antimicrobial stewardship programs and offering an electronic data-tracking system to help monitor the use of certain drugs.

At the University of Wisconsin Hospital and Clinics in Madison, Sarah Bland, senior clinical pharmacist, calls herself the "antibiotic police." Working with an infectious-disease specialist, she uses Premier's software program, called SafetySurveillor, to track the antibiotics prescribed in the 450-bed hospital. The aim is to get doctors to use the narrowest-spectrum antibiotic possible—a drug that is designed to attack only the bacteria causing a specific infection.

Ms. Bland says patients admitted to the hospital or the ER [emergency room] are often prescribed a powerful, broad-spectrum antibiotic such as ciprofloxacin to cover any possible infection. Once lab tests come back with a specific diagnosis, such as a urinary-tract infection that can be treated with a narrow-spectrum drug like amoxicillin, the best course may be to substitute the new drug, she says. Instead, she says, doctors may simply leave the patient on ciprofloxacin or add the second drug.

"Cipro is incredibly potent and active against many different kind of bacteria, but it is something we should have kept in reserve for the most serious infections, and we don't do that," says Ms. Bland. "Every unnecessary dose I avert preserves that drug a little more for the next patient down the line."

Some hospitals have measured tangible benefits. Hunterdon Medical Center in Flemington, N.J., a 178-bed community hospital affiliated with VHA, joined the Bugs and Drugs program in 2006. The hospital developed guidelines for the most commonly overused antibiotics, and routinely tests bacteria from its facility to determine their susceptibility to drugs in its formulary. In a 2007 test, Hunterdon found that 51% of cultures of *Klebsiella pneumoniae*, which causes pneumonia, urinary tract and wound infections, were susceptible to ciprofloxacin, up from 27% a year earlier. Over the period the susceptibility to antibiotics of another infection-causing bacteria, *Pseudomonas aeruginosa*, rose to 79% from 54%.

Pending Legislation

The recent hospital programs come as legislation is pending in Congress to create a federal office of antimicrobial resistance and a public-health network to help detect emerging resistant strains of bacteria before they become a national threat. The National Quality Forum, the leading government advisory body on health-care quality standards, plans to issue revised safety standards for hospitals this fall [2008] including a new requirement that hospitals implement antimicrobial stewardship programs, according to Charles Denham, co-chairman of its Safe Practices group.

Legislation is pending in Congress to create a federal office of antimicrobial resistance.

Hospitals also are under new cost pressures to better manage their antibiotic prescriptions, which account for 30% to 50% of many hospitals' total drug budgets. Medicare announced last summer [2007] that starting [October 2008] it will no longer pay the extra cost of treating some preventable injuries and infections that occur while a patient is in a hospital. The following year, it will add to the list hospital-acquired blood infections and pneumonia acquired on a ventilator. Private insurers including Aetna Inc. and WellPoint Inc. are evaluating their own policies on the issue.

"There is finally recognition by physicians that this is their problem, not just everyone else's," says Neil Fishman, director of the antimicrobial management program at the University of Pennsylvania Medical Center, which other hospitals have used to model their own programs.

A New Role for Doctors

Still, for doctors, it's a new role that can run counter to traditional practices. The programs can pit the desire of doctors to use the most powerful antibiotic for their own patient against medical evidence about the use of such drugs in the general population. The programs also can override doctors' own decisions and force them to answer to pharmacists, who previously merely filled their orders.

At Maine Medical Center in Portland, clinical pharmacist Rob Owens, co-director of the antimicrobial stewardship program, says the program uses a computerized system that requires doctors to answer five questions about the patient before they can order an antibiotic. The system rejects inappropriate antibiotics and automatically orders the correct one, though doctors can override the system under certain circumstances. Dr. Owens says the program helped reverse a trend of rising bacterial resistance at the hospital over a five-year period ended in 2003. Tests showed bacterial susceptibility to certain antibiotics improved by between 20% and 47%, and the hospital has been able to maintain those trends since that time, he says.

Dr. Owens says he examines a list of about 135 patients daily and may find 20 to 40 whose antibiotic therapy he needs to review with physicians. "It takes a little human touch to just tap a doctor on the shoulder and say hey, guys, you may not have seen this lab result, but you happen to have the patient on two drugs that cover the same infection. Maybe two aren't necessary."

Studies at the hospital have shown that when the program was used to prescribe antibiotics, use of the drugs was more appropriate.

"Infectious-disease doctors may only see their individual patient and don't see that in six months you might as well try Holy Water to cure this bug," says Vivien Ng, director of performance improvement at VHA. Once they see data showing that a pattern of resistance is emerging in their hospital to a common antibiotic, "their jaws drop" she says.

The University of Pennsylvania's antibiotic-management team includes infectious-disease doctors, pharmacists and staff from the microbiology lab. The group regularly updates guidelines for antibiotic use at the hospital's Web site. The use of certain antibiotics requires prior approval, and an infectious-disease doctor is on call to arbitrate disagreements.

Hospitals still need to work with doctors from the community and local health officials to get the word out about over-prescribing antibiotics.

Studies at the hospital have shown that when the program was used to prescribe antibiotics, use of the drugs was more appropriate. There also was an increased cure rate for infections, and a reduction in the rate of infections that weren't cured. Over a one-year period, the hospital saved $302,400 on antibiotic costs, $533,000 on infection-related costs and $4.2

million in costs measured from start of intervention in antibiotic therapy to hospital discharge from shorter ICU stays, the hospital says. The program also showed a trend toward decreased emergence of resistance.

Analyzing Patterns

Some VHA member hospitals are working with the University of Florida in Gainesville, which offers a free program to analyze a hospital's patterns of drug resistance and compares these with regional, state or national benchmarks. The program has been used by about 400 hospitals, according to its developer, John Gums, a professor of pharmacy and medicine, who has financed the program with grants from pharmaceutical companies.

But hospital efforts may not be enough, says Robert Pickoff, chief medical officer at New Jersey's Hunterdon Medical Center. He says hospitals still need to work with doctors from the community and local health officials to get the word out about over-prescribing antibiotics. "We interchange patients with doctors in the community all the time, so the expert use of antibiotics has to be followed by everyone," Dr. Pickoff says. "Anyone who doesn't has the potential of breaking the system down and reversing all the progress we've made."

The Government Must Create Economic and Regulatory Incentives for Drug Companies to Develop New Antibiotics

Genetic Engineering & Biotechnology News

Genetic Engineering & Biotechnology News *is a bi-weekly newsletter focusing on the biotechnology industry.*

During the late 1960's, my college roommate suffered a seemingly minor skin infection on a finger, which quickly turned into blood poisoning and resulted in a hip abscess. The infection resolved completely after a few weeks of therapy with a penicillin derivative and repeated aspirations of pus.

That success story is less likely to be repeated today. Especially, if the infection is one contracted in a hospital—in a surgical wound, for example, or in the form of pneumonia—there is a high probability that the bacteria responsible will be resistant to one or more antibiotics.

A High Rate of Resistant Infections

As many as two million patients nationwide contract infections in hospitals each year, and 90,000 die, according to the Centers for Disease Control and Prevention (CDC). The death rate in such cases is alarmingly high, not because the patients initially are gravely ill, but because hospital germs increasingly are resistant to multiple antibiotics.

About 70% of infections are resistant to at least one drug, making them hard to treat. In many cases, we're already out of

Genetic Engineering & Biotechnology News, "Are We Being Outdone by Bacteria? Novel Antibiotics and More Cautious Use of Drugs Needed to Quelch Drug-Resistant Bugs," vol. 26, May 15, 2006. Copyright © 2008 *Genetic Engineering & Biotechnology News*. Reproduced by permission of Mary Ann Liebert, Inc.

good second- or third-line alternatives that are effective, can be administered by mouth, and have few side effects. Hence, we must resort to drugs that are inconvenient to administer or are toxic.

Many of these bad bugs are, however, spreading beyond our hospitals into the greater community.

A future with few effective antibiotics will be treacherous. Also, many of today's routine medical procedures from surgical operations to chemotherapy will be far more dangerous if we permit the bacteria to outwit us.

Antibiotic-resistant pathogens also lead to higher health-care costs because they often require more expensive drugs and extended hospital stays. The total cost to U.S. society is nearly $5 billion annually, according to the Infectious Diseases Society of America.

The trends toward increasing numbers of infections and increasing drug resistance show no sign of abating, and previously unusual bacteria are gaining prominence. An example is Acinetobacter baumannii, outbreaks of which are plaguing hospitals in the U.S., Europe, and elsewhere. It evolves a resistance to multiple antibiotics unusually quickly and also survives on dry surfaces for many weeks.

Many of these bad bugs are, however, spreading beyond our hospitals into the greater community. Given sufficient time and exposure, bacteria use a variety of enormously clever genetic and metabolic tricks to resist any drug we invent.

Staph Developing Resistance

Federal agencies are acutely aware of the importance of this issue. Unless antibiotic resistance problems are detected as they emerge and actions are taken to contain them, the world could be faced with previously treatable diseases that have again become untreatable, as in the days before antibiotics were developed, according to the FDA [U.S. Food and Drug Administration].

Important initiatives are under way by the government and the private sector to promote more sparing and intelligent use of antibiotics.

An example that supports this pessimistic view is our waning ability to treat the common pathogen Staphylococcus aureus, or S. aureus, which causes pustules and abscesses on the skin and can spread to the bloodstream, lungs, brain, bones, or heart, causing severe organ damage and death. Nearly all S. aureus strains have now become resistant to penicillin, and many have become resistant to methicillin and other similar drugs that used to comprise the second line of treatment for S. aureus infections.

Vancomycin was long considered to be the only uniformly effective drug for methicillin-resistant S. aureus. However, a decade ago strains of S. aureus with decreased susceptibility to vancomycin were reported for the first time in Japan and the U.S.

The CDC is concerned about this development, saying, If we are unable to limit the emergence and spread of resistance and to replace drugs like vancomycin as they lose their effectiveness, S. aureus and other similar common bacterial infections may become untreatable, as they were 60 years ago.

The Government Response

To combat this public health emergency, important initiatives are under way by the government and the private sector to promote more sparing and intelligent use of antibiotics.

Regulators and livestock producers are collaborating to reduce the amounts of antibiotics used to prevent disease in livestock. Many HMOs [health maintenance organizations] have adopted policies that restrict antibiotics to infections that seem unequivocally to be caused by bacteria. In other words, patients should not routinely get antibiotics for colds, which are caused not by bacteria, but by viruses. The CDC is conducting a campaign to prevent antibiotic resistance in healthcare centers that consists of four main strategies: prevent infection, diagnose and treat infection, use antimicrobials wisely, and prevent transmission.

Federal officials, however, have paid little attention to the flip side of the problem: the shortage of new antibiotics. Just 20 years ago, approximately a half-dozen new antibiotics would appear on the market each year. Now it's at most one or two.

For decades we've relied largely on new variations on old tricks to combat rapidly evolving pathogens. Most antibiotics in use today are chemically related to earlier ones discovered between 1941 and 1968. During the last 37 years, only two antibiotics with truly novel modes of action have been introduced—Zyvox in 2000 and Cubicin in 2003, the latter used only against skin infections.

BioShield II ... would have created tax incentives for companies that develop new antibiotics and would limit their liability for side effects.

Market forces and regulatory costs have exacerbated the antibiotics drought. Until about a decade ago, all the major pharmaceutical makers had antibacterial research programs. They have dramatically trimmed or eliminated these efforts, however, focusing instead on more lucrative drugs that treat chronic ailments and lifestyle issues. Think Lipitor and Levitra, for example. Whereas antibiotics cure a patient in days, and may not be required again for years, someone with high cholesterol or erectile dysfunction might pop expensive pills every day for decades.

Creating Incentives and Changing Policies

Moreover, drug development has become hugely expensive, with the direct and indirect costs to bring a drug to market now averaging more than $800 million.

We need both legislative and FDA-initiated remedies. In 2005, Senators Joe Lieberman (D-CT) and Orrin Hatch (R-UT) introduced BioShield II, legislation that, if enacted, would have created tax incentives for companies that develop new antibiotics and would limit their liability for side effects, as has been done for vaccines. It would also have extended patents on antibiotics to compensate for time lost while awaiting FDA approval.

The bill's most controversial provision was wild-card exclusivity, which would have allowed a drug company that markets a new antibiotic to extend the patent on any product in its portfolio by up to two years with the approval of federal officials. If Pfizer were to discover a new antibiotic, for example, the company might be granted more time to market Viagra before generic manufacturers were permitted to produce that drug.

Although the wild-card idea offers the best hope of fostering antibiotics research, it was a little too wild in its proposed form. It would have permitted federal officials to grant a wild-card patent extension whenever a pharmaceutical maker developed an antibiotic that met the FDA's broad definition of a new chemical entity. Under this language, if Bayer were to chemically alter its already marketed antibiotic ciprofloxacin (Cipro), for example, the company might qualify for a lucrative patent extension on Levitra, even if the new antibiotic wasn't significantly better than its precursor.

A more appropriate standard would be that in order to qualify for wild-card exclusivity, a drug company's new antibiotic would have to meet FDA's criteria for fast-track designation during development—a product that is intended for the treatment of a serious or life-threatening condition and demonstrates the potential to address unmet medical needs. Thus, a new antibiotic would qualify if it were intended for serious infections and if it were active against bacteria widely resistant to existing antibiotics, if it were more easily administered, or had fewer side effects than alternatives.

If we are to stimulate the development of new antibiotics, other aspects of public policy need attention as well. It has been said that when the FDA sneezes, the pharmaceutical industry gets pneumonia. A chilling example is the delay of an injectable antibiotic called Tigecycline for infections caused by antibiotic-resistant pathogens. Its manufacturer, Wyeth-Ayerst Laboratories, had done two human studies to show that the drug was safe and effective and was planning a third and final one.

Unless we create economic and regulatory incentives for companies to develop antibiotics, it's unlikely that we'll see many more wonder drugs in the near future.

In 2000, however, the FDA changed the rules for measuring efficacy in antibiotics' trials, which required the company to double the number of patients in the trials from 4,000 to 8,000. That made the investment required by Wyeth much greater in both time and money. The drug finally was approved in 2005.

This kind of policy decision has a pernicious ripple effect. As a result [of FDA's change in policy], we've got fewer companies involved in the antibiotic discovery business at a time when antibiotic resistance to existing drugs is becoming more of a problem, according to Robert C. Moellering, Jr., M.D., chairman of the department of medicine at Beth Israel Deaconness Medical Center in Boston.

We need also to adopt the kinds of critical FDA reforms suggested by the Infectious Diseases Society of America. Among them are expediting the publication of updated guidelines for clinical trials of antibiotics, including a clear definition of what constitutes acceptable surrogate markers as endpoints; encouraging imaginative clinical trial designs that lead to a better understanding of antibiotics' efficacy; the exploration of animal models of infection, in vitro technologies, and microbiologic surrogate markers to reduce the number of efficacy studies required; and the FDA's granting of accelerated review status to priority antibiotics.

The two novel antibiotics introduced since 2000 won't be enough to keep rapidly mutating pathogens at bay for long, and once resistance appears, it will spread rapidly. Unless we create economic and regulatory incentives for companies to develop antibiotics, it's unlikely that we'll see many more wonder drugs in the near future. That's something to think about next time you contract bronchitis or are hospitalized with a flesh-eating bacterial infection.

Bold Initiatives Outside the Drug Industry Are Needed to Address the Crisis of Resistant Infections

New York-Presbyterian Hospital

New York-Presbyterian Hospital is a university hospital located in New York City.

The looming threat of bacterial infections resistant to available antibiotics can be averted if industry, regulators, and academics work together in creative new ways, writes Weill Cornell Medical College expert Dr. Carl Nathan in a commentary in the October 21 [2004] *Nature*.

"Despite growing bacterial resistance to existing drugs, antibiotic development in the pharmaceutical industry is steeply declining," warns Dr. Nathan, Chairman of the Department of Microbiology and Immunology at Weill Cornell Medical College and Co-Chair of the Immunology and Microbial Pathogenesis Program at the Weill Cornell Graduate School of Medical Sciences in New York City.

The decline in development of antibiotics for infections prevalent in economically developed regions is merging with the long-standing shortage of antibiotics for infections that mostly afflict less affluent areas. In fact, Dr. Nathan argues that the two crises can best be addressed if they are considered facets of a single problem that has the same causes and potential solutions.

"Government agencies and professional societies have addressed antibiotic resistance, but little has changed," he writes. "We need new approaches."

New York-Presbyterian Hospital, "Bold New Initiatives Are Needed to Address the Crisis of Antibiotic Resistance, According to Weill Cornell Expert," October 18, 2004. Reprinted with permission.

167

Non-Profit Drug Companies and Other Approaches

One approach may involve working with the cooperation of, but outside the regular structure of, the pharmaceutical industry. According to Dr. Nathan, the intense pressure put on the private sector for wide profit margins means drug companies are increasingly forced to drop their traditional pursuit of antibiotic development.

To fill the gap, he supports the creation of "another kind of player on the scene: a not-for-profit drug company," focused on identifying and patenting new drugs and drug combinations overlooked by industry.

This type of non-profit initiative would license its intellectual property "gratis to any company or agency that commits to produce and distribute the resulting drugs on a basis that serves the needs of patients and society," Dr. Nathan writes.

A second innovation involves changing a regulatory system that restricts antibiotic development while encouraging widespread resistance to these drugs, according to Dr. Nathan.

The use of antibiotics in combination is key to their long-term effectiveness, so regulatory changes that encourage manufacturers to test specific drug "synergies" may be crucial, he says. Patent life should also be extended for newly minted antibiotics aimed at novel microbial targets, and "all new antibiotics should be banned from widespread administration to healthy animals," since the use of antibiotics in agriculture remains a prime source of resistance today.

Finally, Dr. Nathan believes scientists and academics must change their approach to antibiotics research. For years, he writes, efforts have focused on a very limited number of microbial targets, "producing almost nothing but variants of older antibiotics." Now, he says, "the well has gone dry."

Thanks to the recent explosion of knowledge in genetics and cellular biology, researchers now have a multitude of largely unexplored "points of vulnerability" at which to target new antibiotic drugs, Dr. Nathan points out.

Diagnostics can and must be improved, he says, and scientists must also move away from developing drugs that work against a broad spectrum of pathogens, since this encourages microbial resistance. Instead, he says, "it is medically preferable, and will preserve the utility of the drugs longer, if antibiotics are highly specific, so that each one is used less often."

"Is it hopelessly unrealistic to envision not-for-profit companies, a smart regulatory environment, and fresh scientific approaches to antibiotic development?" Dr. Nathan asks. Perhaps not: He points out that not-for-profit entities—like the Bill and Melinda Gates Foundation, and the Medicines for Malaria Venture—are already having a significant impact on new drug discovery.

In the end, he says, the search for new, effective antibiotics cannot be allowed to fail.

"All sectors of society, including the pharmaceutical industry, have a major stake in the control of infectious diseases," Dr. Nathan writes, "not only for medical reasons but also for global economic development and security."

The Public and Private Sectors Need to Support Pro-Research Legislation

David Fleming and Jeffrey S. Duchin

David Fleming, M.D., is director and health officer for Public Health in Seattle and King County in the state of Washington. Jeffrey S. Duchin, M.D., is chief of the communicable disease epidemiology and immunization section of the department.

Recent news describing serious infections caused by methicillin-resistant Staph aureus (MRSA) has focused needed attention on the problem of drug-resistant infections. However, inaccurate information has led to unnecessary fear and inappropriate actions. It's time to reassess the threat and what we can do about it.

The MRSA Crisis

Staph aureus are common bacteria that live on the skin or in the nose of approximately 30 percent of people, usually without causing any symptoms. MRSA are Staph aureus that are resistant to the drug methicillin and related antibiotics. About 1 percent of the U.S. population carries MRSA on their body without becoming ill. Both MRSA and non-methicillin-resistant Staph aureus cause skin infections such as boils, ulcers and abscesses and can also cause serious invasive infections, primarily in hospitalized patients. Recently, MRSA has been increasing as a cause of infections in the community, including among people who are generally healthy.

The majority of MRSA infections are uncomplicated skin infections that can be treated with other available antibiotics. Less commonly, the infections are severe and even fatal. MRSA

David Fleming and Jeffrey S. Duchin, "Re-Examine the MRSA Threat," *Seattle Post-Intelligencer*, November 21, 2007. Reproduced by permission.

170

is passed from person to person through close skin-to-skin contact, and infections also can occur through contaminated items and surfaces.

The good news is that there are simple steps we can take to reduce the risk of MRSA infections: good hand and personal hygiene, prompt medical care for skin infections, keeping wounds covered, not sharing personal items such as towels and shavers, and avoiding close skin-to-skin contact with people who have wounds. Because MRSA pneumonia can follow influenza, getting vaccinated against the flu is a good idea. Disinfection of surfaces contaminated by any Staph aureus, including MRSA, is also advised, but extraordinary disinfection measures in schools and workplaces are generally not necessary.

MRSA is one example of a larger problem because of antibiotic resistant bacteria. Over the years, antibiotics have saved millions of lives and eased patients' suffering. But increasingly, bacteria have developed resistance to antibiotics, making infections difficult and at times impossible to treat.

The pipeline of new antibiotics is drying up because of a marked decrease in industry research and development.

Infections caused by resistant bacteria can strike anyone. They lead to higher health care costs, often requiring more expensive drugs and extended hospital stays. The total cost to U.S. society nears a staggering $5 billion annually. This trend of drug resistance shows no signs of slowing, and the prospect is real that effective antibiotics may not be available to treat seriously ill patients in the near future.

Responding to the Threat

Unfortunately, the public and private sectors appear to have been lulled into a false sense of security based on past successes. The pipeline of new antibiotics is drying up because of a marked decrease in industry research and development. Major pharmaceutical companies are losing interest in the antibiotics market because these drugs are not as profitable as drugs that treat other conditions.

[The STAAR Act] would bolster needed research, improve critical data collection, [and] promote more appropriate use of existing antibiotics.

Can anything be done about the increasing threat? We need to educate physicians, patients and parents about the appropriate use of antibiotics, emphasize the importance of basic infection control measures, develop safer alternatives to the current use of antibiotics in agriculture and stimulate new antibiotic drug development.

One more important thing can be done right now with the help of elected officials in Congress. The Strategies to Address Antimicrobial Resistance [STAAR] Act, HR3697, is a bipartisan bill that has the potential to save lives by strengthening the response to increasingly resistant infectious pathogens. It would bolster needed research, improve critical data collection, promote more appropriate use of existing antibiotics and support the leadership needed to direct those efforts. [H.R.3697 was introduced in the House on September 27, 2007, and in the Senate (S.2313) on November 6, 2007. S.2313 was referred to the Committee on Health, Education, Labor, and Pensions, and H.R.3697 to the Committee on Energy and Commerce Subcommittee on Health. The STAAR Act was not enacted by the 110th Congress by the end of 2008, but the Infectious Diseases Society of America is pushing for reintroduction in the 111th Congress in 2009.]

Drug-resistant infections are everybody's problem. To solve it, we need to take action in our communities and by supporting national efforts such as the STAAR Act to fight drug-resistant infections.

New Approaches Are Needed to Combat Drug-Resistant Bacteria

Sean S. Kardar

Sean S. Kardar is a graduate student in the molecular and systems pharmacology program at Emory University in Atlanta, Georgia.

The repeated emergence of antibiotic-resistant bacterial strains is a problem that has long plagued public health. Bacteria have always possessed the ability to protect themselves from naturally occurring antibiotics by acquiring resistance through the exchange of genetic material with other bacteria. In the last two decades, however, the problem has escalated as the prevalence of antibiotic-resistant bacteria has increased and multi-drug-resistant strains have emerged in many species that cause disease in humans.

Antibiotics have proven to be a major asset in the fight against infectious bacteria.

The prognosis is grim. There are no treatments available for infections caused by many of the antibiotic-resistant bacteria, and resistance to commonly used antibiotics is steadily increasing. In fact, no class of drugs with a novel mode of action has been developed since the introduction of nalidixic acid in 1962. Alternative methods to combat antibiotic-resistant bacteria are needed and scientists have begun to search for antimicrobial drugs in vertebrates, invertebrates, and even bacteria and fungi in Earth's most extreme environments—from Yellowstone National Park's hot springs to the 120,000-year-old glaciers in Greenland.

Sean S. Kardar, "Antibiotic Resistance: New Approaches to a Historical Problem," ActionBioscience.org, March 2005. Reproduced by permission.

Historical Timeline of Antibiotics

Antibiotics have proven to be a major asset in the fight against infectious bacteria.

- Louis Pasteur unknowingly described the first antibiotic in 1877 when he observed that certain bacteria release substances that kill other bacteria.

- In 1909, Paul Ehrlich discovered arsphenamine (Salvarsan), an arsenic compound that kills Treponema palladium, the bacterium causing the sexually transmitted disease, syphilis.

- In 1928 Alexander Fleming discovered that a mold inhibited the growth of staphylococcal bacteria and named the substance it produced "penicillin" (possibly Pasteur's unknown substance).

- It was not until 1940 that Howard Florey and Ernst Chain isolated the active ingredient in Fleming's mold.

- With wide-scale production of penicillin, the use of antibiotics increased, leading to an average eight-year increase in human life span between 1944 and 1972. Unfortunately, many bacterial species continued to survive penicillin treatment due to their resistance mechanisms.

Current Status of Resistant Bacteria

There is an alarming rise in the occurrence of antimicrobial resistance. For example:

- *Staphylococcus aureus* is a prevalent bacterium carried by humans that can cause a number of problems, from mild skin infections to serious diseases including food poisoning, wound infections, pneumonia, and toxic shock syndrome. The World Health Organization

(WHO) recently reported that more than 95% of *S. aureus* worldwide is resistant to penicillin, and 60% to its derivative methicillin.

- Today in the U.S. more than 20% of all enterococcal infections, that is, infections caused by intestinal colonizing bacteria in the genus *Enterococcus* are resistant to vancomycin, once considered the antibiotic of last resort.

Antibiotics are the third largest selling class of drugs, with an annual market between $7 billion and $22 billion. Current estimates suggest that of this expenditure $4 billion to $5 billion results from antibiotic-resistant bacteria. Although the resistance problem continues to mount, pharmaceutical companies have made little progress in the development of new bactericidal drugs. Consequently, surveillance programs for early detection of multi-drug resistant bacteria, such as Sentry, have been implemented. Supported by the University of Iowa and private donations, Sentry conducts microbial surveys in 33 nations on 5 continents, gathering over 50,000 samples of various infectious bacteria. Other programs include England's Alexander Project and programs directed by the Centers for Disease Control and Prevention (CDC) and WHO. Their goal is to explore short- and long-term strategies to combat antibiotic resistance.

Causes of Antibiotic Resistance

For many years it was believed that antibiotic resistance was only caused by the failure of prescribed drug regimens. It is now accepted that human errors also contribute to the development of antibiotic-resistant bacteria.

- *Misuse of antibiotics* occurs in medicine, agriculture, and household products. Common examples include erroneous antibiotic prescriptions for nonbacterial infections and the addition of antibiotics to livestock feed and cleaning agents, which have helped create a reservoir of antibiotic-resistant bacteria.

- *Anomalous combinations* have perpetuated drug-resistant microbes. For example, one study on Rhesus monkeys reports that mercury in dental amalgam fillings fostered a 61% increase in antibiotic-resistant bacteria. Upon removal of the amalgam fillings, drug-resistant bacteria dropped 58%. In another example, *S. aureus* was shown to acquire vancomycin resistance genes through cohabitation with the vancomycin-resistant bacteria, *Enterococcus faecalis*, in the wound of a hospitalized patient. Through mechanisms of genetic exchange between bacterial species, the mere coexistence of these two particular bacteria helped to bring about drug resistance in *S. aureus*.

- *Enhanced transmission of resistance factors*, or the increased efficiency with which resistance genes are exchanged, is another important way that antibiotic resistance is perpetuated. Factors that contribute to enhanced transmission include the survival of patients with chronic disease, an increased number of immunosuppressed individuals, substandard hospital hygiene, more international travel, and budget cuts in health care administration.

- *The reservoir hypothesis* suggests that antibiotic-resistant bacteria have evolved because of the selective pressures applied by antibiotic drugs; moreover, the hypothesis states that each antibiotic has a threshold level that is required to induce and maintain antibiotic resistance. After a decline in the populations of susceptible bacteria from antibiotic treatment, naturally resistant bacteria begin to thrive, creating a reservoir of antibiotic-resistant bacteria.

New Era of Antimicrobial Therapeutics

It is a fact that selection of multi-drug-resistant bacteria has occurred throughout history. Unfortunately, however, drug-resistant bacteria have been met with antibiotics that are nothing more than recapitulations of earlier drugs. There has been an urgent need for new avenues of therapeutic treatment, and a new era of prophalytic (preventative) treatment has begun. Here the most plausible approaches are described:

- bacterial interference

- bacteriophage therapy

- bacterial vaccines

- cationic peptides

- cyclic D,L-a-peptides

Bacterial Interference: Bacterial interference, also known as bacteriotherapy, is the practice of deliberately inoculating hosts with nonpathogenic (commensal) bacteria to prevent infection by pathogenic strains. To establish an infection and propagate disease, pathogenic bacteria must find nutrients and attachment sites (adhesion receptors). Infection by pathogenic bacteria is prevented by commensal bacteria, which compete with pathogenic bacteria for nutrients and adhesion receptors or spur attack through secretion of antimicrobial compounds.

This treatment has had promising results in infections of the gut, urogenital tract, and wound sites. The major advantage of using bacteria in a positive way to benefit health, known as "probiotic" usage, is that infection is avoided without stimulating the host's immune system and decreases selection for antibiotic resistance. Understanding how bacterial species compete, an essential criterion for research, has been known for at least 20 years but its practical application has yet to be realized.

177

Bacteriophage Therapy: Bacteriophages (commonly called "phages") are viruses that infect bacteria and were recognized as early as 1896 as natural killers of bacteria. Bacteriophages take over the host's protein-making machinery, directing the host bacteria to make viral proteins of their own. Therapeutically, bacteriophages were used as a prophylaxis against cholera, typhoid fever, and dysentery from the 1920s to the early 1940s. The practice was abruptly stopped when synthetic antibiotics were introduced after World War II. Now that there is a plethora of multi-drug-resistant bacteria, bacteriophage therapy once again has become of keen interest.

Bacteriophage therapy is quite attractive for the following reasons:

- phage particles are narrow spectrum agents, which means they possess an inherent mechanism to not only infect bacteria but specific strains

- other pathogens may be targeted through manipulation of phage DNA

- exponential growth and natural mutational ability make bacteriophages great candidates for thwarting bacterial resistance

Bacterial Vaccines: Development of bacterial vaccines has become an increasingly popular idea with the advent of complete genomic sequencing and the understanding of virulence regulatory mechanisms.

- Bacterial genomics allows scientists to scan an entire bacterial genome for specific sequences that may be used to stimulate a protective immune response against specific bacterial strains. This approach expedites the drug discovery process and, more importantly, provides a more rational, target-based approach.

- The best targets are essential bacterial genes that are common to many species of bacteria, which code for proteins with the ability to gain accesses through lipid membranes, and possess no homology to human genes.

- Regulatory genes that control virulence protein production are excellent vaccine candidates for priming the human immune system or inhibiting virulence production.

- Bacterial genomics can also detect conserved sequences from bacterial species and strains worldwide. This technology will inevitably yield superior clinical vaccine candidates.

Cationic Peptides: These diverse peptides are natural compounds that posses both hydrophobic and hydrophilic characteristics, which means portions of the molecule are water avoiding or water loving. Cationic peptides are found throughout nature in the immune systems of bacteria, plants, invertebrates, and vertebrates.

These peptides are not the usual synthetic drugs encountered in pharmaceutical drug design; however, they do exhibit antibacterial effects. Cationic peptides have several mechanisms of action, all of which involve interaction with the bacterial cell membrane leading to cell death. From a therapeutic standpoint, these proteins have great promise, as they have co-evolved with commensal bacteria yet have maintained the ability to target pathogenic bacteria.

Antibiotic resistance is a continually evolving and dangerous problem that requires immediate attention.

Cyclic D,L-a-peptides: Unlike cationic peptides, cyclic D,L-a-peptides are synthetic and amphipathic (molecules having both water loving and water hating characteristics) cell membrane disruptors. As the name implies these peptides are cyclic in nature and are composed of alternating D and L amino acids. Cyclic D,L-a-peptides are engineered to target gram-positive and negative membranes (not mammalian cell membranes). In contrast to any other known class of peptides, these peptides can self-assemble into flat ring shaped confirmation-forming structures known as nanotubes, which specifically target and puncture bacterial cell membranes resulting in rapid cell death.

Time to Act

Antibiotic resistance is a continually evolving and dangerous problem that requires immediate attention as well as future planning to impede a global health crisis. Is it not time to seriously consider other methods for which current antibiotic therapies are ineffective and therefore prolong sickness, treatment, and even sometimes result in mortality? Many feel these new alternatives, such as those discussed in this article, are not mainstream. I would agree, but since the efficacy of current therapies is waning and conventional antibiotics are a temporary fix to bacterial multi-drug resistance society must look elsewhere. If the reservoir hypothesis is true, as most scientists agree, then curbing drug usage to prevent resistant bacteria should be key. Although this viewpoint is highly debated, it holds some merit. Bacteria thrive on mutations and removal of selective pressures should slow mutational rates. Indeed, the alternative methods mentioned have begun to target the pathogen and not the organism.

In addition to current research efforts, the world's health organizations, such as WHO, CDC, and the Food and Drug Administration (FDA) are building better monitoring systems to detect rising numbers of multi-drug-resistant bacteria. It is not enough, however, physicians and patients must do their part by understanding the ease with which bacteria develop resistance and the consequences of antibiotic misuse.

Organizations to Contact

The editors have compiled the following list of organizations concerned with the issues debated in this book. The descriptions are derived from materials provided by the organizations. All have publications or information available for interested readers. The list was compiled on the date of publication of the present volume; the information provided here may change. Readers need to remember that many organizations take several weeks or longer to respond to inquiries.

Alliance for the Prudent Use of Antibiotics (APUA)
75 Kneeland St., Boston, MA   02111-1901
(617)636-0966 • fax: (617)636-3999
e-mail: apua@tufts.edu
Web site: www.tufts.edu/med/apua

The Alliance for the Prudent Use of Antibiotics is a nonprofit global organization founded in 1981 to contain antibiotic resistance and improve antibiotic effectiveness. APUA's mission is to strengthen society's defenses against infectious disease by promoting appropriate antimicrobial access and use and controlling antimicrobial resistance on a worldwide basis. The APUA Web site is an excellent source of information on the issue of antibiotic resistance for consumers, health care practitioners, and researchers.

Center for Interdisciplinary Research to Reduce Antimicrobial Resistance (CIRAR)
Columbia University School of Nursing
630 est 168th St., Box 6, New York, NY   10032
(212)305-0723 • fax: (212)305-0722
e-mail: el123@columbia.edu
Web site: www.nursing.hs.columbia.edu/CIRAR

The Center for Interdisciplinary Research to Reduce Antimicrobial Resistance, initially funded in 2004 by a planning grant from the National Center for Research Resources of the National Institutes of Health, is now an established, ongoing research center supported by the Columbia University School of Nursing. CIRAR prepares biomedical researchers to conduct interdisciplinary research on the prevention and control of antimicrobial resistance. The CIRAR Web site lists various on-line scientific publications relating to the issue of antibiotic resistance.

Centers for Disease Control and Prevention (CDC)
1600 Clifton Rd., Atlanta, GA   30333
(800)232-4636 • fax: (770)488-4760
e-mail: cdcinfo@cdc.gov
Web site: www.cdc.gov

The Centers for Disease Control and Prevention, part of the U.S. Department of Health and Human Services, is the primary federal agency for conducting and supporting public health activities in the United States. The CDC works to ensure the health of Americans; as part of this effort, the CDC operates programs to prevent antibiotic resistance in health care settings, to research the level of resistance in the United States, and to educate the public about antibiotic resistance. The CDC Web site contains a wealth of information about antibiotic resistance as well as links to congressional testimony, various organizations working on the issue, and other resources.

Keep Antibiotics Working
P.O. Box 14590, Chicago, IL   60614
(773)525-4952
Web site: www.keepantibioticsworking.com

Keep Antibiotics Working is a coalition of health, consumer, agricultural, environmental, humane, and other advocacy groups dedicated to eliminating the inappropriate use of antibiotics in food animals. Among the materials available on its Web site are fact sheets, such as "Antibiotic Resistance—An

Emerging Public Health Crisis" and "Antibiotic Resistance and Animal Agriculture." Other resources include press releases, consumer information, and links to reports published by other organizations.

Microbe World
1752 N St. NW, Washington, D.C. 20036-2904
(202)737-3600
e-mail: microbe@asmusa.org
Web site: www.microbeworld.org

Microbe World is a Web site created by the American Society for Microbiology to educate the public about the profession and issues related to the study of microbiology. A search of the Web site's "In the News" topic leads to information about antibiotic resistance, and the site also contains a link to *Microbe*, the society's monthly news magazine.

MRSA Resources Support Forum
Web site: www.forum.mrsaresources.com/viewtopic.php?t=672

MRSA Resources Support Forum is a support forum for people who have been affected by Methicillin-resistant *Staphylococcus aureus* (MRSA) and other so-called superbugs.

National Foundation for Infectious Diseases (NFID)
4733 Bethesda Ave., Suite 750, Bethesda, Maryland 20814
(301)656-0003 • fax: (301)907-0878
e-mail: info@nfid.org
Web Site: www.nfid.org

The National Foundation for Infectious Diseases is a non-profit, tax-exempt organization founded in 1973 and dedicated to educating the public and health care professionals about the causes, treatment, and prevention of infectious diseases. NFID supports research that will lead to a better understanding of the causes, cures, and prevention of infectious diseases. A search of the NFID Web site for antibiotic resistance produces a list of materials relating to this topic.

National Institute of Allergy and Infectious Diseases (NIAID)

NIAID Office of Communications and Government Relations
6610 Rockledge Dr., MSC 6612, Bethesda, MD   20892-6612
(301)402-1663 • fax: (301)402-0120
e-mail: niaidnews@niaid.nih.gov
Web site: www3.niaid.nih.gov

The National Institute of Allergy and Infectious Diseases, part of the National Institutes of Health, conducts and supports basic and applied research to better understand, treat, and ultimately prevent infectious, immunologic, and allergic diseases. NIAID research has led to new therapies, vaccines, diagnostic tests, and other technologies that have improved the health of millions of people in the United States and around the world. A search of the NIAID Web site for antibiotic resistance yields fact sheets and various other materials on the subject.

Sustainable Table

215 Lexington Ave., Suite 1001, New York, NY   10016
(212)991-1930 • fax: (212)726-9160
e-mail: info@sustainabletable.org
Web site: www.sustainabletable.org

Sustainable Table is a Web site created in 2003 by the nonprofit organization GRACE to help consumers understand the problems with our food supply and offer viable solutions and alternatives. Sustainable Table is home to the *Eat Well Guide*, an online directory of sustainable products in the United States and Canada, and several critically acclaimed movies about sustainable living. The Web site's "Antibiotics" section presents an informative summary of the problem of antibiotic resistance and sustainable alternatives.

Union of Concerned Scientists (UCS)

2 Brattle Square, Cambridge, MA   02238-9105
(617)547-5552 • fax: (617)864-9405

Web site: www.ucsusa.org

The Union of Concerned Scientists is a science-based non-profit organization devoted to working for a healthy environment and a safer world. UCS combines independent scientific research and citizen action to develop innovative, practical solutions and to secure responsible changes in government policy, corporate practices, and consumer choices. UCS's Food and Agriculture Program focuses on reducing the use of antibiotics in food animals, and clicking on this topic leads the reader to several articles about antibiotic resistance, including for example, "The Mounting Scientific Case Against Animal Use of Antibiotics" and "Statement on Hogging It!: Estimates of Antimicrobial Abuse in Livestock."

Bibliography

Books

Carlos F. Amabile-Cuevas — *Antimicrobial Resistance in Bacteria.* Boca Raton, FL: Taylor & Francis, 2006.

Gerald N. Callahan — *Infection: The Uninvited Universe.* New York: St. Martin's Press, 2006.

I.W. Fong and Karl Drlica — *Antimicrobial Resistance and Implications for the 21st Century.* New York: Springer, 2007.

Connie Goldsmith — *Superbugs Strike Back: When Antibiotics Fail.* Breckenridge, CO: Twenty-First Century Books, 2006.

Ian M. Gould and Jos W.M. van der Meer — *Antibiotic Policies: Fighting Resistance.* New York: Springer, 2007.

William R. Jarvis — *Bennett and Brachman's Hospital Infections.* Philadelphia: Lippincott Williams & Wilkins, 2007.

Ramanan Laxminarayan, Anup Malani, David Howard, and David L. Smith — *Extending the Cure: Policy Responses to the Growing Threat of Antibiotic Resistance.* Washington, D.C.: RFF Press, 2007.

Stuart B. Levy · *The Antibiotic Paradox: How the Misuse of Antibiotics Destroys Their Curative Powers.* New York: Da Capo Press, 2002.

Abigail A. Salyers and Dixie D. Whitt · *Revenge of the Microbes: How Bacterial Resistance Is Undermining the Antibiotic Miracle.* Herndon, VA: ASM Press, 2005.

Michael A. Schmidt · *Beyond Antibiotics: Strategies for Living in a World of Emerging Infections and Antibiotic-Resistant Bacteria.* Berkley, CA: North Atlantic Books, 2009.

Michael Shnayerson · *The Killers Within: The Deadly Rise of Drug-Resistant Bacteria.* Boston: Back Bay Books, 2003.

Jeannie Mitchell Thomas · *License To Kill.* Kansas City, MO: Leathers Publishing, 2006.

Thomasine E. Lewis Tilden · *Help! What's Eating My Flesh?: Runaway Staph and Strep Infections!* London: Franklin Watts, 2007.

Christopher Walsh · *Antibiotics: Actions, Origins, Resistance.* Herndon, VA: ASM Press, 2003.

Richard G. Wax, Kim Lewis, Abigail Salyers, and Harry Taber · *Bacterial Resistance to Antimicrobials.* Boca Raton, FL: CRC, 2007.

Debbie Weston   *Infection Prevention and Control: Theory and Practice for Healthcare Professionals.* Chichester, England: Wiley-Interscience, 2008.

Periodicals

The A to Z of Materials   "Nanotechnology Help Boost Antibiotics in Combating Resistant Infections," Oct. 13, 2008. www.azom.com/News.asp?NewsID=14073.

Alicia Ault   "More Action Needed on MRSA," *Skin & Allergy News*, vol. 39, Mar. 2008.

CBS News   "Super-Resistant Superbugs: Lesley Stahl Reports On Drug-Resistant Infections," May 2, 2004. www.cbsnews.com/stories/2004/04/30/60minutes/main614935.shtml.

Centers for Disease Control and Prevention   "CDC Estimates 94,000 Invasive Drug-Resistant Staph Infections Occurred in the U.S. in 2005: Study Establishes Baseline for MRSA Infection Estimates," Oct. 16, 2007. www.cdc.gov/media/pressrel/2007/r071016.htm.

The Economist (US)   "Riding Piggyback; Drug-Resistant Infections," vol. 385, no. 8557, Dec. 1, 2007.

Erik Goldman   "MRSA Showing No Mercy in Skin Infections," *Internal Medicine News*, vol. 40, no. 19, Oct. 1, 2007.

Marc Kaufman "Worries Rise Over Effect of Antibiotics in Animal Feed: Humans Seen Vulnerable to Drug-Resistant Germs," *The Washington Post*, Mar. 17, 2000.

Lindsay Lyon "Report Spells Out How to Stop Hospital Infections," *U.S. News & World Report*, Apr. 17, 2008.

Medical News Today "MRSA Linked to Rising Number of Severe Bone Infections, Health Complications in Children," July 1, 2008. www.medicalnewstoday.com/ articles/113440.php.

Modern Healthcare "MRSA, Other Staph Infections Are Now Endemic," vol. 37, no. 48, Dec. 3, 2007.

Carl Nathan "Antibiotics at the Crossroads," *Nature*, vol. 431, Oct. 21, 2004.

Norml "Pot Compounds Reduce Multi-Drug Resistant Infections, Study Says Cannabinoids Show 'Exceptional' Antibacterial Activity Against MRSA," Aug. 28, 2008. http://norml.org/ index.cfm?Group_ID=7687.

Micheal Pollan "The Way We Live Now: Our Decrepit Food Factories," *The New York Times Magazine*, Dec. 16, 2007. www.nytimes.com/2007/12/16/ magazine/16wwln-ledet.html?_r= 2&scp=1&sq=%22Our%20Decrepit% 20Food%20Factories%22&st=cse& oref =slogin&oref=slogin.

The Real Truth   "Drug-Resistant Staph Infections Up
                          Sevenfold," June 4, 2007.
                          www.realtruth.org/news/
                          070604-002-health.html.

Red Orbit   "Higher Incidence of Drug-Resistant
                          Staph Infection in Gay Men," Jan. 15,
                          2008. http://www.redorbit.com/
                          news/health/1216581/higher_incidence_
                          of_drugresistant_staph _
                          infection_in_gay_men/index.html.

Reuters   "Hospital Testing for Drug-Resistant
                          Infections Dramatically Lowers
                          Mortality Rates . . . ," Mar. 4, 2008.
                          www.reuters.com/article/pressRelease/
                          idUS192107+04-Mar-2008+PRN20080304.

Antony Savvas   "NHS Equips Wards with
                          Infection-Resistant Keyboards,"
                          ComputerWeekly.com, Apr. 21, 2008.
                          www.computerweekly.com/
                          Articles/2008/04/28/230459/
                          nhs-equips-wards-with-infection-
                          resistant-keyboards.htm.

ScienceDaily   "US Hospitals Report Infections
                          Increasing in Frequency and Cost,"
                          Sept. 26, 2007. www.sciencedaily.com/
                          releases/2007/09/070925130019.htm.

Science Daily   "New Approach May Render
                          Disease-Causing Staph Harmless,"
                          Feb. 16, 2008. www.sciencedaily.com/
                          releases/2008/02/080214144409.htm.

Science Daily   "Alligator Blood May Put the Bite on
                       Antibiotic-Resistant Infections," Apr.
                       7, 2008. www.sciencedaily.com/
                       releases/2008/04/080407074556.htm.

Science Daily   "New Antibiotic Beats Superbugs at
                       Their Own Game," July 7, 2008.
                       www.sciencedaily.com/releases/2008/
                       07/080703113648.htm.

Nancy Shute   "4 Ways to Avoid MRSA Infections
                       in Kids," *U.S. News & World Report*,
                       Sept. 8, 2008.

Katie Thomas   "Experts Say Staph Is Common
                       Problem for Athletes," *The New York
                       Times*, Oct. 24, 2008.
                       www.nytimes.com/2008/10/25/
                       sports/football/25staph.html?partner=
                       rssnyt&emc=rss.

University of   "'Superbug' Infections More Than
Florida News   Doubled in Hospitals, Study Finds,"
                       Nov. 30, 2007. http://news.ufl.edu/
                       2007/11/30/mrsa-infections.

S. Williams   "Superbug: What Makes One
                       Bacterium So Deadly," *Science News*,
                       vol. 172, no. 20, Nov. 17, 2007.

Index

A

Abbott Laboratories, 116, 129

Aborted-infection Immunization, 53

Academy of Veterinary Consultants, 87

Acinetobacter, 114–115

Agency for Healthcare Research and Quality (AHRQ), 140

AHRQ (Agency for Healthcare Research and Quality), 140

Allen, Arthur, 31–35

Alliance for Prudent Use of Antibiotics (APUA), 66

American Association of Bovine Practitioners, 87

American College of Physicians, 104

American Public Health Association (APHA), 21, 147

American Society for Microbiology, 117

American Veterinary Medical Association, 87

Aminoglycosides, 75

Amoxicillin, 21

Animal agriculture
    antibiotics, 60–98, 142–145
    cattle industry, 85–86
    environmental routes, 145–146
    Europe, 93
    fluoroquinolones, 87
    food routes, 145
    government oversight, 85–87
    Guidance for Industry Part 152, 87
    human infections link, 145–148
    on-farm quality assurance programs, 98
    public health threat, 146–147
    resistance management, 86–87
    risk assessments, 87
    safety, 98

Anthrax, 32, 101, 113

Antibiotic resistance, 62–64
    anomalous combinations, 176
    causes, 26–28, 175–176
    enhanced transmission of resistance factors, 176
    genetics, 89, 93, 143–144
    global spread, 26
    human factor, 28–30
    misuse of antibiotics, 175–176
    reasons, 109
    reservoir hypothesis, 176
    threat, 22–23
    veterinary antibiotics, 56
    zoonotic origin, 70–71, 76–78, 91–93

Antibiotic-resistant bacteria (ARB), 70–71, 74–75

Antibiotics
    alternative methods, 173
    appropriate use, 23–24, 28–29
    children, 121–122
    conservative treatment, 122–123
    controls, restrictions, 28
    dangers, 120–121
    decreasing strength, 112–113
    discovery, 27